Men's Health
Advisor 1995

MEN'S HEALTH ADVISOR 1995

EDITED BY
MICHAEL LAFAVORE

Men's Health Magazine

Rodale Press, Emmaus, Pennsylvania

"Sailing Away" by Chris Byron. Copyright © 1994 by Chris Byron. Reprinted by permission.

"Going to the Sex Therapist" by Frank Pittman, M.D. Copyright © 1993 by Frank Pittman, M.D. Reprinted by permission.

"Love Potions and Spells" by Roger McElvey. Copyright © 1993 by Roger McElvey. Reprinted by permission.

ISBN 0–87596–252–1
ISSN 1060–9407

Distributed in the book trade by St. Martin's Press

2 4 6 8 10 9 7 5 3 1   hardcover

OUR MISSION

We publish books that empower people's lives.

RODALE 🐝 BOOKS

Men's Health Advisor 1995 Editorial and Design Staff

EXECUTIVE EDITOR, *Men's Health* Magazine: Michael Lafavore

SENIOR EDITOR: Russell Wild

GROUP VICE-PRESIDENT: Mark Bricklin

PROJECT COORDINATOR: Dominick Bosco

BOOK DESIGNER: Alfred Zelcer, Charles Beasley

COVER DESIGNER: Stan Green

COVER PHOTOGRAPHER: Mark Hanouer/Onyx

ILLUSTRATOR: Gary Hovland

STUDIO MANAGER: Joe Golden

TECHNICAL ARTIST: David Q. Pryor

MANAGING EDITOR, *Men's Health* Magazine: Steven Slon

RESEARCH EDITOR, *Men's Health* Magazine: Melissa Gotthardt

COPY EDITOR: John D. Reeser

OFFICE STAFF: Roberta Mulliner, Julie Kehs, Bernadette Sauerwine, Mary Lou Stephen

OFFICE MANAGER, *Men's Health* Magazine: Susan Campbell

Men's Health Books

EDITOR-IN-CHIEF, RODALE BOOKS: Bill Gottlieb

EXECUTIVE EDITOR: Debora A. Tkac

ART DIRECTOR: Jane Colby Knutila

RESEARCH MANAGER: Ann Gossy Yermish

COPY MANAGER: Lisa D. Andruscavage

NOTICE

This book is intended as a reference volume only, not as a medical manual. The information given here is designed to help you make informed decisions about your health. It is not intended as a substitute for any treatment that may have been prescribed by your doctor. If you suspect that you have a medical problem, we urge you to seek competent medical help.

Contents

10 ASK *MEN'S HEALTH*

Introduction

HAS ANYONE KICKED YOUR TIRES LATELY?

IS IT REALLY TRUE THAT we men take better care of our cars than we do our own bodies?

Perhaps. But if it is true, things are certainly changing. The overwhelming response to *Men's Health* magazine and the past years' *Men's Health Advisor*s tells me that we are taking better care of ourselves.

Maybe we're more interested in better health because as much fun as a car can be, our bodies can be an even richer source of pleasure and fulfillment.

Or maybe it's just because it costs more to fix our bodies when they break!

Either way, there are a few things you need to know if you're going to take better care of yourself, things like . . . well, how healthy are you? . . . and what are your specific trouble spots that need more work than the other areas?

Sort of like the well-placed kick you deliver to the tire of a car you're thinking of buying . . . or that all-important spin around the block to check power, cornering and the rattles in the suspension. Not to mention the radio.

Well, the first chapter of this *Men's Health Advisor 1995* fulfills this need. "What's Your True Age?" will tell you just what state your body is in and your probable life expectancy.

But don't worry, we don't treat you like a ton of steel and plastic in a used car lot. We tell you how to improve your score, with specific instructions for your problem areas.

And that's just the first chapter. Page after page of the *Men's Health Advisor 1995* will provide you with information you need to feel younger and stronger, and to live healthier and happier lives—at any age.

It's not impossible—in fact, it's not even very difficult. The *Men's Health Advisor 1995* is dedicated to the proposition that you can keep yourself strong now and forever without driving yourself nuts with rules and exhausting yourself with exercise. The experts say that driving your body hard is not what's going to make you strong and healthy. On the contrary: Moderate amounts of exercise deliver the greatest benefit.

So go ahead, kick your tires. Take yourself for a spin around the block. As good as it is, it can get better. And the *Men's Health Advisor 1995* is here to help.

Michael Lafavore
Executive Editor
Men's Health Magazine

Part 1

HOW A MAN
STAYS YOUNG

What's Your True Age?

A few key actions can boost your life expectancy by 15 years. Take this test for a measure of your true age.

• • • • • • • • • • • • • • • • • • •

YOU CAN THINK OF LIFE as the ultimate distance sport, in which the goal is to put your body through its paces with as much aplomb and ease of movement as possible. The better your condition, the less difficult the course will be and the longer you'll last. Which is to say that when you're going the distance, the key to success is endurance. The question here is, do you have what it takes to outlast the next guy?

To answer that, you need to look at how well you've been training. Normal life expectancy is based on averages among people who have very good health habits and very bad ones, notes Paul Terry, Ph.D., author of *It's Your Body: An Up-to-Date Guide to Healthy Living and Preventing Medical Problems.* "If your habits are good," he says, "you'll add years above what's considered normal."

According to this view, all of us have the potential to live considerably longer than the male average of 71.2 years if only we will reverse (or at least slow down) the damage we do ourselves through various choices and behaviors. Researchers at Duke University in Durham, North Carolina, have calculated that by taking charge of key life-shortening behaviors, you can boost your life expectancy by 15 years. "What you're really doing," Terry says, "is getting years back."

As Robert F. Allen, Ph.D., writes in his book *Lifegain,* "While there's no sure way to calculate exact life expectancy even with computers, there are certain guidelines that can give you rough estimates." And, he says, getting such an estimate can be a valuable first step in changing those life-shortening habits most of us have.

QUIZ YOURSELF

With some help from experts, we've formulated our own quiz to help you figure out where you stand. (Hey, if life insurance companies can do it, so can we.) Now take out a pencil, good luck, and may the last man win.

To start

As you go through the test, keep a running total of your score. At the end, you'll add or subtract this tally from a life expectancy that's average for men your age.

Family History

Your greatest health risks start with your genes: The big man killers—heart disease, prostate cancer and colon cancer—are all inheritable. Having a history of any of them at least doubles your risk of getting them yourself. In the case of prostate cancer, family history is the only major risk factor.

Score

1. Grandparents lived to at least 80? Add 1 for each instance.

2. Mother or father lived that long? Add 3 for each.

3. Mother or father died of a heart attack or stroke before age 50? Subtract 4 for each.

4. Any immediate family member (parent, sibling, grandparent) has or has had cancer or a heart condition or diabetes since childhood? Subtract 3 for each instance.

5. Any family member die of the above problems before age 60? Subtract 2 for each.

6. Any immediate family member die of prostate cancer, colon cancer or any other natural cause before age 60? Subtract 1 for each.

To improve your score

Even men who are prone to specific diseases can reverse their risks by fighting the factors that contribute to the problems. Eating a diet rich in fruits and vegetables, for example, lowers your risk of both colon cancer and cardiovascular disease. Regular doctor's exams allow for early detection and vastly increase your chances of surviving prostate and other cancers.

Exercise

Because exercise has been proven so important to health, the American Heart Association added sedentary lifestyle to the cholesterol/weight/blood pressure trinity of risk factors for heart disease.

Research shows that a man with through-the-roof cholesterol and blood pressure levels who's in great physical shape is actually less at risk of dying young than a man with lower cholesterol readings who's inactive. As further evidence of this tradeoff, one study finds that active older men have four times fewer strokes than inactive peers. Less dramatic but significant results are also reported for cancer, particularly the colorectal variety.

Score

1. Exercise aerobically for at least 30 minutes three or more times a week? Add 2.

2. Play sports or do light physical activities like yard work once or twice a week? Add 1.

3. Almost never exercise? Subtract 2.

To improve your score

If you don't exercise now, start. Even a 20-minute-a-day walking program can improve your overall fitness. Realize, however, that after a point, more isn't necessarily better. Experts say that moderate amounts of activity deliver the greatest benefits.

Cholesterol

Between ages 45 and 64, men have almost *four times* as many heart attacks as women, and high cholesterol is a critical risk factor. And some research even suggests high cholesterol is a risk factor for prostate cancer.

Score

1. Total cholesterol has always been 200 or less? Add 4.

2. Total cholesterol now 200 or less, but was once between 240 and 299? Add 3.

3. Total cholesterol now 200 or less, but was once 300 or more? Add 2.

4. Total cholesterol now at 240 to 299? Subtract 1.

5. Total cholesterol now above 300? Subtract 2.

To improve your score

The obvious course is to lower saturated fat and dietary cholesterol. But it's just as important to stay active. In one large study, people who walked for 2½ to 4 hours a week had half the risk of high cholesterol that sedentary people had.

Alcohol

As a potentially addictive drug, alcohol is ripe for abuse; when abused, it ruins the liver and pickles the brain. Still, studies suggest that the occasional drink is not just harmless, it may actually boost longevity.

Score

1. Drink moderately (no more than two beers, two glasses of wine, two shots of whiskey a day on average), but not to the point of drunkenness? Add 2.

2. Abstain totally from alcohol? Add 1.

3. Regularly drink until intoxicated? Subtract 6.

To improve your score

If you don't drink, we're not suggesting that you go out and start. Rather, the key is getting help if you have a problem. Alcoholics Anonymous is a proven success, but there are other alternative organizations as well. Check your local newspaper and telephone directory for groups like Rational Recovery or Secular Organizations for Sobriety.

Regular Doctor's Exams

The biggest benefit of checkups lies in warding off premature death from either prostate or colon cancer. Testing is especially important after age 40, when these problems are most likely to develop. A basic checkup involves a digital-rectal exam and a look at your colon with a flexible tool called a sigmoidoscope.

Score

1. Have an annual physical exam? Add 1.

2. Have a proctological exam every other year after age 40? Add 2.

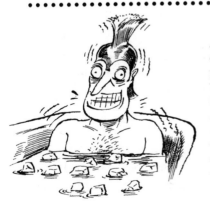

Have a Cold One

A warm bath may mellow you out, but a cold one revs up your body. In research at the Thrombosis Research Institute in London, cold baths increased disease-fighting white blood cells, improved circulation and boosted testosterone for the Spartans who took them regularly.

To improve your score

After age 50, also get a prostate-specific antigen blood test, which can detect signs of prostate cancer that your doctor can't.

Diet

What you put into your body has a proven bearing on your chances of getting heart disease and certain types of cancer. Fatty foods, for example, can raise cholesterol, boost blood pressure and contribute to cancer of the colon—not to mention make you fat. The dietary prime directive is to get no more than 30 percent, and preferably less than 25 percent, of calories from fat. This automatically puts more fruits and vegetables on your plate. Fruits and vegetables naturally supply life-extending nutrients, particularly vitamins C, E and beta-carotene, which have been shown to reduce risk for a wide range of health problems. Plus, there is evidence that they protect against heart disease as well. In one study, men who got more than 50 milligrams of vitamin C (about half the amount in an eight-ounce glass of orange juice) had half the death rate of men who got less than 50 milligrams.

Score

1. Get five or more helpings of fruits and vegetables daily? Add 5.

2. Eat a lot of high-fat foods like red meat, fried foods and snack items, but try to balance these with plenty of fruits and vegetables? Add 1.

3. Eat a lot of high-fat foods; rarely if ever eat fruits and vegetables? Subtract 4.

To improve your score

Many experts say that the official guidelines for adequate intake of vitamins C, E and beta-carotene are too low, so it's worth taking a multivitamin supplement in addition to maintaining a good diet.

Smoking

Among risk factors you can do something about, "smoking overwhelms everything else," says Daniel Nixon, M.D., vice-president for professional education at the American Cancer Society. It plays a role in just about every major health problem men face. Smoking is the leading cause of lung cancer and may play a role in prostate and colon cancer as well. It also causes high blood pressure. In light of all this, it's not surprising that death rates for smokers over age 65 are roughly twice as high as for nonsmokers the same age.

Score
1. Never smoked? Add 2.

2. Quit five or more years ago? Add 1.

3. Smoke less than half a pack a day? Subtract 1.

4. Smoke one-half to one pack a day? Subtract 2.

5. Smoke one to two packs a day? Subtract 6.

6. Smoke more than two packs a day? Subtract 10.

7. Smoke marijuana once a week or more? Subtract 1.

To improve your score
Obviously, quitting makes a huge difference. Within five to ten years of quitting, lung cancer risk reverts to near normal. One proven strategy for quitting is to get your nicotine fix in ways other than smoking. Nicotine gum is one way, and the nicotine patches introduced last year are another. For further information on how to quit, contact the National Cancer Institute at 1-800-422-6237.

• •

Put the Squeeze on Hypertension

Squeezing a grip-strengthener, grabbing a tennis ball or just pressing your palms against each other a few times a week may help lower your blood pressure. In one study, people with mild high blood pressure (hypertension) who did this kind of exercise for four two-minute sessions three times a week for eight weeks cut blood pressure levels by up to 15 points. Why the technique works is not clearly understood, but researchers theorize that tensing the muscles for short periods may alter hormone levels that influence blood pressure. Light weight training has also been shown to reduce blood pressure. But gripping too hard or holding any grip too long can raise your blood pressure. If you have high blood pressure, check with your doctor before trying this gripping regimen.

Blood Pressure

More than a third of men have high blood pressure. In effect, this reading is a measure of how hard your heart has to work to pump blood through your body. And if your heart works too hard, well, that's not good: High blood pressure is a proven cause of both stroke and heart disease. The reading is expressed as two numbers—anything close to 120/80 is considered normal—with the second number, diastolic blood pressure, being the primary yardstick.

Score

1. Diastolic blood pressure has always been 88 or lower? Add 3.

2. Diastolic blood pressure is 88 or lower, but was once between 89 and 104? Add 2.

3. Diastolic blood pressure is 88 or lower, but was once 105 or higher? Add 1.

4. Diastolic blood pressure is between 90 and 104? Subtract 1.

5. Diastolic blood pressure is above 104? Subtract 2.

To improve your score

Light exercise is the key. Studies show that regular brisk walks can bring the blood pressure numbers down and decrease your risk of stroke and heart attack by up to 56 percent and 37 percent, respectively. Persistent high blood pressure requires medication.

Stress

Even though anxiety can't be precisely measured, emotional pressure is associated with a wide range of debilitating problems, particularly heart disease. One study, for example, finds that middle-age men who describe themselves as highly stressed have almost twice the rate of coronary artery disease as men who rate their stress low.

Score

1. Best description of you is easygoing and relaxed? Add 3.

2. Best description of you is aggressive, intense, easily angered? Subtract 3.

3. Demanding job with little say over how things get done? Subtract 2.

4. Four or more years of college? Add 3.

5. One to three years of college? Add 2.

6. High school only? Add 1.

To improve your score

One of the worst offenders here is frustration with work, particularly work of a high-demand, low-control nature. Education may give you an edge, though: Some research indicates that educated men tend to be in-control managers while less-educated peers tend to do the take-orders grunt work.

Obesity

Being more than a few pounds overweight can shave years off your life. Obesity is related to high cholesterol, high blood pressure and adult-onset diabetes. And research suggests these relationships are especially strong in men younger than age 45. There's also evidence that being overweight puts you at higher risk for certain types of cancer.

Ideal weight is a factor of your height and frame size. To determine your frame size, bend your forearm upward at a 90-degree angle, keeping your fingers straight and turning the inside of your wrist toward your body. Place the thumb and index finger of your other hand on the two prominent bones on each side of your elbow. Measure the space between your fingers. Below are the measurements for a man with a medium build. If the measurement is smaller or larger, so is your frame.

● ●

Height	**Elbow Breadth**
5′2″–5′3″	2½″–2⅞″
5′4″–5′7″	2⅝″–2⅞″
5′8″–5′11″	2¾″–3″
6′0″–6′3″	2¾″–3¼″
6′4″	2⅞″–3¼″

● ●

Now that you know your frame size, find your ideal weight in the chart on page 10.

Height	FRAME Small	Medium	Large
5′2″	128–134	131–141	138–150
5′3″	130–136	133–143	140–153
5′4″	132–138	135–145	142–156
5′5″	134–140	137–148	144–160
5′6″	136–142	139–151	146–164
5′7″	138–145	142–154	149–168
5′8″	140–148	145–157	152–172
5′9″	142–151	148–160	155–176
5′10″	144–154	151–163	158–180
5′11″	146–157	154–166	161–184
6′0″	149–160	157–170	164–188
6′1″	152–164	160–174	168–192
6′2″	155–168	164–178	172–197
6′3″	158–172	167–182	176–202
6′4″	162–176	171–187	181–207

SOURCE: Metropolitan Life Insurance Company

Score

1. Have always been within 5 percent of your ideal weight? Add 2.

2. Currently within 5 percent of ideal weight, but were once more than 30 percent over? Add 1.

3. Have always been from 5 to 30 percent overweight? Subtract 1.

4. Weight has fluctuated by more than ten pounds several times since high school? Subtract 2.

5. Have always been more than 30 percent overweight? Subtract 4.

To improve your score

The best weight–loss plan combines a low-fat diet with modest exercise for gradual changes. Avoid crash dieting, as question four suggests. Studies find that losing weight rapidly and then gaining it back (which is likely with quick-loss plans) puts you at even higher risk for coronary artery disease than being just moderately overweight.

- Begin with age 71, which is the average life expectancy for men.

- Next, adjust for your current age. If you're over 29, add one point for every decade mark you've passed beyond 29 (i.e., if you're 30, add one; if you're 40, add two; and so on).

- Now total your score from the questions above. Add or subtract it on line d below. The final total is your estimated life expectancy.

a) Average life expectancy: *71*

b) Age adjustment:

c) Adjusted total (a+b):

d) Score from questions above:_____

e) Total (estimated life expectancy):_____

One final point: Good health habits deliver not only longer life but *better* life. Even if you don't end up beating the odds, taking corrective measures will assure you of being a whole lot happier and more comfortable in your later years.

—Richard Laliberte

The Male Body, an Owner's Manual

What self-respecting man can let a valuable machine go to pot? It's time to take better care of your body than you do your car.

• • • • • • • • • • • • • • • • • • •

FOR EVERY MAN THERE IS a machine. Some guys love computers, some moon over motorcycles. There are chain-saw nuts and ultralight freaks, steam engine hounds and mixer masters. Here we are in the middle of a post-industrial revolution and otherwise normal men are out there hanging their hearts on machines. They are part of our biology: To men, machines are the souvenirs of common sense, the concrete icon of our ideal selves. Something profound happens to a man when he pushes the "go" button and the big wheel goes around, ticks a gear, turns a spring and makes the whole thing say "howdy" in tool talk.

For most men, of course, the machine of choice is a car. Women in the know understand completely that the way to most men's hearts is through the passenger-side door of their man's favorite ride. Men love cars. They go fast when we can't, and they look good when we don't. Every guy with a driver's license has known that magic moment coming out of a tight turn when he becomes his machine, pops his clutch and burns rubber down a long straightaway.

So why don't we take as much care with the other important machine in our lives—the body—as we do with our cars? What is it that cars have that bodies don't?

That's easy: decent rust protection and an owner's manual. You do the undercoating. We'll provide the manual: Follow the maintenance advice here, and you'll stay on the road for years to come.

BONES

Bones are the framework on which the rest of the body is hung. Structural integrity is crucial for providing overall support, withstanding stresses or collisions and ensuring freedom of movement.

Maintenance. Even after major repairs from breaks or fractures, bones generally require little maintenance over the body's lifetime, but their functional usefulness can be greatly extended by two basic procedures.

1. Add calcium regularly. Keep bones well-supplied with the stuff from which they're built.

Reason: Women have big problems with brittle bones for the usual hormonal reasons, but one-third of the hips that break annually from the weakening effects of osteoporosis are male hips, according to Sydney Lou Bonnick, M.D., osteoporosis researcher at Texas Women's University in Denton.

Men do a good job of getting regular calcium supplies until about age 25. That's when a man's drinking choices begin shifting to coffee, soda and alcohol in place of one of the best dietary sources of calcium, milk. As a result, the average man gets about 25 percent less calcium than recommended.

It takes very little milk to keep bones stocked with raw material. You need about 1,000 milligrams of calcium a day but are probably about 250 short. It is highly advised that you drink one eight-ounce glass of skim milk per day, which provides about 350 milligrams.

2. Observe manufacturer's minimum strength levels.

Reason: Bones in bodies that do physical work are strong bones. Men who toil at desks and are not active during a normal day should exercise regularly by lifting weights. While bones also get stronger from weight-bearing activities such as walking, running, tennis or basketball, weight training is best. A full-body weight regimen has the potential to add bone, while aerobic exercise serves primarily to maintain existing bone. A second reason is that during a weight workout it is easier to target specifically the hips and back, the areas most vulnerable to bone loss.

Tools. One 310-pound barbell set and bench. Cost: about $300.

Troubleshooting. You can make yourself bad to the bone by wearing stupid shoes, having a lousy bite or otherwise making your skeleton do something it wasn't intended to do. Unexplained aches and pains could be a sign of abnormal stress on the bones—don't let them go unattended.

HEART

The heart is your power plant, vital for transporting oxygen and nutrients throughout the body. Keeping it running smoothly requires a high level of efficiency throughout the entire vascular system.

Maintenance. The heart is strong but it works ceaselessly. It is prone to breakdown if it is not diligently maintained over time. Keeping risk factors in check can be accomplished through three basic steps.

1. Don't use cheap fuel. Your best diet is a mix that's rich in carbohydrates, low in protein and low in fat. Realistic proportions are 60 percent carbohydrates, 10 to 15 percent protein and 25 to 30 percent fat. But you don't have to worry about the numbers if you center your meals around fruits, vegetables and grains (including pasta). Keep your intake of meat, poultry and seafood between four and six ounces a day. Avoid add-on fats like butter or oil.

Reason: A low intake of fat prevents cholesterol sludge buildup and keeps weight and blood pressure down. Also, recent studies suggest that a diet rich in antioxidants, a class of nutrients that includes vitamin C and beta-carotene, protects against heart disease. In one study, men who ate high levels of vitamin C were 42 percent less likely to die of heart disease than men who didn't. In another, taking the amount of beta-carotene equivalent to two carrots a day lowered heart attack risk by about 45 percent in male physicians with heart disease.

2. Blow out the pipes. Be physically active, preferably with a program of regular aerobic exercise, such as walking, running, swimming or bicycling.

Reason: Exercise is so important to maintaining heart health that the American Heart Association has deemed the lack of it to be a risk factor on a par with smoking, high blood pressure or cholesterol problems. By the way, it's not necessary to exercise at a high intensity. Regular aerobic exercise—such as brisk walking for 30 minutes three times a week—can do the job.

3. Use proper additives. A further step to consider under doctor's guidance is to take regular doses of aspirin.

Reason: Aspirin has been shown to reduce heart attack risk substantially, even in quantities ten times lower than the amount found in a standard 325-milligram tablet. Many doctors recommend taking low-dose aspirin tablets of 81 milligrams daily, or a standard dose every other day. Ask your physician about what may be appropriate for you.

Tools. One good pair of cross-training shoes. One gym membership (optional).

Troubleshooting. If your heart goes on the blink, try running down this little checklist.

Smoking. Most smokers die of heart attacks, not cancer, says Carl Lavie, M.D., medical co-director of cardiac rehabilitation and prevention at Oschner Heart and Vascular Institute in New Orleans. Smoking contributes to obstruction of arteries and formation of blood clots at blockage sites. Quitting substantially reduces risk within six to nine months, according to Dr. Lavie.

Weight. Being overweight makes the heart work harder and increases the danger from most other major risk factors. To determine your ideal weight, start with a base of 105 pounds, then add 6 pounds for each inch of height above 5 feet. Example: The ideal weight for a man measuring 5-foot-11 would be 105 plus 66 (11 extra inches times 6 pounds per inch), which comes out to 171. If you have a large frame, add another 10 percent, which in this case would raise you to 188.

Blood pressure. This is a measure of how forceful the blood pushes on the walls of the arteries. It's also the level of pressure that the heart's pumping must exceed as it pumps blood into circulation. Blood pressure is expressed as a measure of two numbers: the top number or systolic pressure (during a heartbeat) and the bottom number or diastolic pressure (between beats). A blood pressure reading above 140/90 is

• •

Old Wonder Drug

Expensive anti-inflammatory drugs have all but replaced aspirin for treatment of arthritis, supposedly because they produce fewer side effects. But in fact, says a group of researchers at Stanford University School of Medicine, the opposite is true. In a study of arthritis patients, the researchers found that aspirin produced far fewer side effects, such as stomach pain, than five other arthritis drugs. They say that previous studies used aspirin dosages that were much higher than those used in actual practice.

considered too high and carries with it an increased risk of stroke, heart attack and other vascular diseases. Just a 15 unit increase in the diastolic blood pressure, say from a normal of 80 to an abnormal of 95, can double all these risks says Robert DiBianco, M.D., associate clinical professor of medicine at Georgetown University School of Medicine in Washington, D.C., and director of cardiology research at Washington Adventist Hospital in Takoma Park, Maryland. So, a few extra pounds, a little more salt and less exercise might just have a big effect on your long-range health. Sometimes that's all it takes to increase your blood pressure.

Cholesterol. There are two kinds, good and bad. The bad kind (LDL) deposits fatty plaque on artery walls, leading to blockages. The good kind (HDL) helps keep arteries clear. Your key concern is not total cholesterol but the ratio between total and HDL levels. To determine this, divide total cholesterol by HDL. You're in good shape if the result is 4.5 or below.

Big Troubleshooting. Tightness in the chest. If pain is severe; radiates from the chest to the shoulders, neck, arms or jaw; or is accompanied by dizziness, sweating, nausea or breathlessness, you could be having a heart attack. Dial 911, call for help, but don't panic.

SKIN

A shabby or prematurely aged exterior can tarnish the luster of a well-tuned body.

Maintenance. The skin is the only major organ of the body that's directly exposed to the outside, which makes it easy to monitor its condition but also makes it vulnerable to hazards that aren't problems for the rest of your body.

1. Keep it in the shade. The best way to avoid skin damage is to wear sunscreen with a sun protection factor (SPF) of 15 or more. Dermatologist Ivor Caro, M.D., associate clinical professor of medicine at the University of Washington in Seattle, suggests daily application of one of the new skin moisturizers that double as sunscreens. They're not thick like regular sunscreens, don't clog pores and are often unscented. As a plus, they'll keep your skin from drying.

2. Buff the finish. The only other skin matter to be routinely concerned about is shaving, which can be tough on the face. To make the going less tough, soften skin with soap and warm water before shaving. You may have thought that's what shaving creams and gels do, but their job is to help the blade glide smoothly over the skin. As for technique, *follow the growth of the beard,* which means down the cheeks and up the neck. It's true you'll shave closer against the grain, but you'll also be more prone to irritation. The reason: If hairs are cut below the surface, they may become ingrown and produce tender red bumps, a condition called pseudofolliculitis.

Tools. One tube of moisturizer with sunscreen of SPF 15 included.

Troubleshooting. If your skin develops a kind of reptilian sheen, you're cruising for a carcinogenic bruising. In fact, over the long haul, the main danger to skin, both in terms of appearance and general upkeep, is sun exposure. Ultraviolet radiation accelerates the aging process, leading to the premature development of lines, wrinkles and leathery texture, says Dr. Caro. It's also the primary cause of skin cancer, the most common type of cancer but highly curable if caught early.

Big Troubleshooting. Moles that change texture or grow larger, darker or more irregular may indicate skin cancer, as may sores that don't heal or persistently recur.

BRAIN

It's the on-board computer that runs the whole machine, both the parts you think about and the parts you don't. And as with other components, it can deteriorate with age if not looked after.

Maintenance. It was once assumed an adult brain couldn't change either physically or chemically. Now, however, studies suggest that improvement is possible, that you can think more clearly, more quickly, more flexibly—and prolong these abilities into your later years. "Any time you work the brain, there's a change," says Robert Dustman, Ph.D., who researches the subject as a career scientist at the Veteran's Administration Medical Center in Salt Lake City. "That's what learning is."

1. Work the body to work the brain. In rats, physical activity makes chemical transmitters in the brain work better. In people, one of Dr. Dustman's studies found that four months of daily walking improved mental agility in 55- to 75-year-olds. Another found that highly fit people do better on tests of brain power than sedentary people. Dr. Dustman speculates that if you do any kind of exercise to increase blood and oxygen flow to the brain, you'll be mentally quicker.

2. Change the channel. Rats who live in cages that are visually interesting and outfitted with play equipment and companion rats have bigger, more complex brains than rats who live in dull isolation, says Dr. Dustman. In a study of older people, those who played video games had faster reaction times (on a test that had nothing to do with the games) than those who just watched movies on TV. Bottom line: Dr. Dustman advises that we try things we haven't done before and spend free time on pursuits that engage the mind, such as games, creative play with children or reading.

Tools. One *New York Times* crossword puzzle or equivalent, taken daily.

Troubleshooting. Feeling stupid? Down in the dumps? Depression and temporary idiocy are obvious signs of either adolescence or fatigue. On the other hand, never dismiss difficulties that suggest a potential problem: weakness or numbness, difficulty talking to or understanding others, visual problems, dizziness. All are possible signs of stroke.

NERVOUS SYSTEM

In a sense, the brain isn't confined to the head but branches throughout the body via the spinal cord and the peripheral nerves. They are the body's wiring.

Maintenance. The biggest threat to the nervous system (aside from paralyzing injury) is stroke. When a brain artery becomes blocked or ruptures, the brain cells it feeds die, and the body parts controlled by those cells stop working. Proper maintenance of the heart will help ward off stroke, but there's an additional preventive step that's also worthwhile, says Alexander Reeves, M.D., chairman of the neurology section at Dartmouth-Hitchcock Medical Center in Hanover, New Hampshire: *Take supplements of vitamin E.*

In studies, a high intake of vitamin E (about 100 international units per day) has been shown to reduce incidence of heart attack by almost 40 percent. "Whether it prevents stroke is not yet clear, but the probability is that it does," Dr. Reeves says. It's thought that vitamin E makes clot-forming platelets in blood less sticky and less liable to clot.

Tools. Vitamin E is difficult to get enough of in the diet because many prime sources, such as nuts and oils, are high in fat and will clog up your arteries if you eat too much. Experts recommend taking supplements.

Troubleshooting. Nothing like a stroke to really alert you to the dangers of high blood pressure and stroke. The evil, wicked part is that most strokes occur without warning. One day you're walking down the street, and the next day you're lying in it. Hence, there's often no trouble to shoot until it's already all over you. Prevention, as they say, is the best medicine.

LUNGS

Lungs are necessarily delicate, to allow free passage of the body's vital gases: oxygen (for energy) and carbon dioxide (waste). Other parts of the respiratory system, such as the nose and bronchial passages, provide filtration to keep out unwanted particles and organisms and air-conditioning to make sure air is humidified and brought to body temperature before reaching the lungs.

Maintenance. Breathe in. Breathe out. Repeat.

Do this a lot, and when you can, do it deeply. Regular aerobic exercise trains muscles to use oxygen more efficiently, so you don't get so easily winded.

Troubleshooting. Threats to the lungs tend to come from outside.

1. Cooties. Of particular concern are bacteria and viruses, which thrive in moist, warm surroundings, and air pollution, which irritates the lungs, leaving them more susceptible to infections and more sensitive to allergens.

The best tactic for staving off damage from common viral invaders is to get an annual influenza vaccine. A bout with the flu can result in lasting lung damage and even death if it progresses to pneumonia. Studies also show that reducing stress may make you less susceptible to colds and other respiratory infections.

2. Smoke. One of the most significant types of air pollution is cigarette smoke, even when it's someone else's. Breathing secondary or sidestream smoke directly (before it dissipates) is actually worse than taking a drag from a cigarette, because much of the smoke is unfiltered and contains higher levels of toxins like tar and ammonia, says Alfred Munzer, M.D., president of the American Lung Association. Where smoke is impossible to avoid, Dr. Munzer recommends that you seek a well-ventilated place, opening a window, if possible.

3. Smog. As for outdoor pollution, when city air is bad, limit activities outdoors and confine exercise to early morning or evening, when levels of traffic-related and industrial pollutants are lowest.

Big Troubleshooting. If you have a cough that lasts for more than one to two weeks, especially if phlegm is produced, you could have pneumonia or bronchitis.

MUSCLES

They didn't call the 1965 Pontiac GTO a muscle car for nothing. Muscle makes the machine go.

Maintenance. Muscle maintenance is one part conditioning and one part injury avoidance. Both goals are accomplished by routinely exercising muscles, which reduces risk of injury by making them stronger.

Best preventive maintenance: First, warm up. Second, stretch. "People often think a stretch and a warm-up are the same thing, and they're not," says New York Giants team physician Allan Levy, M.D., author of *The Sports Injury Handbook: Professional Advice for Amateur Athletes.* What's needed for your warm-up is any activity that makes you break into a slight sweat, raising body temperature and making muscles more flexible and responsive to stretching.

Troubleshooting. You forgot to warm up and stretch? Here's what can happen.

1. Overuse injuries. Soreness is the hallmark. "Don't work through a pain," Dr. Levy says. "Mild injuries can become disabling if they're not rested or treated early enough." To treat sore muscles, do more stretches to prevent tightness. Start by applying heat to loosen tight muscles. After stretching, apply ice to reduce swelling. Dr. Levy recommends filling resealable storage bags with a mixture of ice cubes and water, which keeps the bags' temperature at an even 32 degrees. "That way you don't have to worry about frostbite," he says. Practical benefit: You can hold it in place with an elastic bandage and go about other business.

2. Muscle pulls. Here, muscle fibers are stretched too far. Typically, pulls occur in the hamstrings and calves for men who do sports that require propulsive leg movement, such as basketball, and in the back, neck and shoulders for men who do sports involving rotating motions, such as golf, softball and tennis. Pulled muscles need a few days' rest, says Dr. Levy.

Big Troubleshooting. Mystery pain. You can't always know what it means on the basis of how it feels. Any knucklehead knows that if you work out a long-lazy muscle, it's going to ache later. That's not a mystery. A mystery is when you work out a leg muscle but your kidneys start aching. Any new, unfamiliar pain is your body's way of saying, "Look at me!", and it needs prompt medical attention.

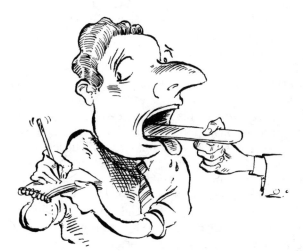

Recall Notice

It might be a good idea to take some notes at your next doctor's appointment. In a recent survey of 1,751 patients, recall of their doctors' advice was as low as 22 percent only a few months after their checkups. Advice about medication was remembered best, while advice about diet and exercise was most commonly forgotten.

SEX ORGANS

You can physically survive without sex organs, but who'd want to? Preserving the sexual apparatus for some men is the whole point of maintaining the rest of the body. And, in fact, following upkeep advice for the rest of the body will do a good job of keeping you sexually primed.

Maintenance. Strengthening the pelvic floor muscles can help maintain erections and control ejaculations. Here's what it takes: Kegels. To do them, squeeze the same muscles you would use to shut off the flow of urine. Relax. Begin doing 5 or 10 of these a day and gradually add more until you're doing up to 50. There's also some evidence that having sex or masturbating regularly keeps your sperm and testes in good working order.

Troubleshooting. Men are vulnerable to a number of problems affecting sex organs. Most can be prevented or fixed through vigilance and regular checkups. Specifically:

1. Prostate cancer. This is the second most lethal cancer in men. In its earliest and most curable stages, it causes no symptoms, making screening vital. The American Cancer Society recommends that men, beginning at age 40, receive annual checkups including a digital-rectal exam and, beginning at age 50, a prostate-specific antigen blood test, both of which are needed for accurate diagnosis of cancer. If you have a family history of the disease or are African American, get both starting at age 40.

2. Testicular cancer. This problem tends to hit earlier than prostate cancer, usually in the twenties. Cure rates for testicular cancer are above 90 percent, but it can still be lethal if left undetected. After puberty, all men should self-examine the testicles monthly, says Kenneth Goldberg, M.D., author of *How Men Can Live as Long as Women.* It's best done in the shower, where heat makes the testicles descend farther from the body. Roll each testicle slowly between your thumb and forefinger. If you feel any lumps or bumps, see a doctor.

3. Prostate enlargement. This one is less lethal, but troublesome for most men at some point, usually after age 40. The prostate surrounds the tube through which urine exits; as the gland grows bigger, it increases the pressure on this tube. Symptoms include needing to urinate more, not being able to go when nature calls and having decreased flow. The aggravations of minor enlargement, such as loss of sleep because of bathroom jaunts, can be alleviated by simple measures like avoiding liquids several hours before bedtime. More advanced problems may require a kind of Roto-Rooter surgery to relieve pressure on the urinary tube.

4. *Impotence.* It's estimated that up to 15 million American men are impotent. And we're not talking about the occasional inability to get an erection that happens to all of us at some time or another. Eighty to 90 percent of true impotence problems are physical in nature, primarily from vascular disease, according to Boston University urologist Irwin Goldstein, M.D., author of *The Potent Male.* The trick is to remember that what's good for your heart is good for your penis and act accordingly. See "Heart" on page 14 for more information.

—*Richard Laliberte*

Build a Stronger Brain

The difference between piercing wisdom and mushy thinking has nothing to do with luck or good genes. Here are 15 steps to help you get smarter.

• • • • • • • • • • • • • • • • • • •

I AM LOSING MY MIND.

I was certain of it the other day. I pulled up to a gas pump and the attendant said, "Your tank's on the other side." So I drove around the island, and, of course, the gas tank was still on the far side of the car.

My brain skipped tracks again that night at dinner. I asked a waitress if she had any wine without steroids. *Sulfites* is what I meant to say, the preservative. I'm starting to sound like my father. Once, on a trip to Dallas, he asked a cab driver to take him to the Ayatollah. He meant the Anatole Hotel. Now, a little mushy thinking can be forgiven in a man of 65, but I'm 32.

Brain drain. Senility. It's easy to believe that these are as certain as wrinkles, a slower 40-yard dash and, um, something else. But are they? Actually, the answer is no. While it does take a little longer for us to process information and learn new tasks as we age, there's plenty of brain power left to carry us to a fruitful old age. "Rapid thought drops off early—you won't see a 70-year-old test pilot—but it's not unusual for a 70-year-old judge to be as wise as ever," says Richard C. Mohs, Ph.D., memory researcher and director of the psychology division at Mount Sinai Medical Center in New York City.

The exciting news is that neuroscientists believe the difference between piercing wisdom and mushy thinking isn't a matter of luck or heredity. Though it's a new area of research, early studies indicate that the brain, like a muscle, seems to get stronger with use. Here's the latest on clearing the occasional fuzziness we experience in middle age and ensuring that we stay sharp well into our eighties.

Get straight Bs. Be sure you get your share of B vitamins, which play important roles in brain function. Some studies suggest that elderly people with significant B-vitamin deficiencies may develop cognitive problems. Vitamin B_6, found in whole wheat, oats, tuna and bananas, may be the most crucial B of all. Dutch researchers gave 38 healthy men in their seventies 20 milligrams of B_6 daily for 12 weeks. At the end of the study, the B_6 patients performed better on tests of their long-term memories than a control group given a placebo. In another Dutch study, doctors found that healthy people with lower blood levels of vitamin B_{12} did not perform as well on a complex test of color identification as people with higher levels.

Hit the books. Keeping yourself intellectually challenged can strengthen your brain and help keep you mentally quick, research suggests. Examining the brains of 20 deceased adults, researchers at the University of California, Los Angeles Brain Research Institute found an anatomical change that reflected how well-educated and mentally active subjects were. Those with college educations who remained mentally challenged throughout life had up to 40 percent longer *dendrites* than those who had less than a high school education and led mentally sedentary lives. *Dendrites* are branchlike parts of nerve cells that bring in information and help promote sophisticated processing. In theory, the more dendrites you have, the more information you can receive and understand.

A sheepskin alone, however, doesn't ensure that you'll always weigh in heavy on the dendrite scale. Even a rocket scientist, if he spends too much of his free time watching *American Gladiators,* could very well experience brain drain, says Bob Jacobs, Ph.D., principal author of the UCLA study.

Jog your noggin. Regular, moderate aerobic exercise may improve our ability to do two things at once, such as carry on a conversation while driving a car. This is a critical mental skill that is known to erode slowly as we age. In a University of Illinois study, formerly sedentary 62- to 74-year-olds did hourlong aerobic workouts in a swimming pool three times a week for ten weeks. Before and after the study, they were tested on their understanding of simultaneous auditory and visual signals. On average, the group scored 30 percent higher after completing the exercise program. Study leader and psychology professor Art Kramer, Ph.D., speculates that exercise may increase the flow of oxygen-carrying blood to the brain. Others point out that increased blood flow also brings in more glucose, which is the brain's fuel, essential to clear thinking.

· ·

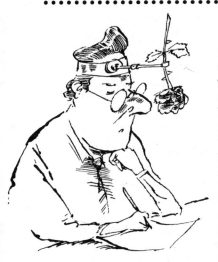

Smell the Roses

If you're looking to boost your brain power, try taking some time to smell the roses. Studies at the Smell and Taste Treatment and Research Foundation in Chicago suggest that flowery odors may help your brain function better. Subjects were able to complete puzzles 17 percent faster if they were exposed to a flowery odor during an experiment. Researchers say the scent may work by relaxing you or improving your mood.

Keep the pressure down. Controlling high blood pressure could help you maintain a healthy mind. One study suggests that years of high blood pressure (hypertension) may actually rob you of brain tissue. Using magnetic resonance imaging, researchers looked at the brains of 35 men between the ages of 51 and 80—18 with high blood pressure (but otherwise healthy) and 17 completely healthy. The result: The men with hypertension showed a significant loss of the white-matter type of tissue that acts as the wiring for the brain. Such tissue loss, "in time, may express itself in problems with memory, language and finding your way around," says Declan Murphy, M.D., senior fellow at the National Institute on Aging in Bethesda, Maryland.

In a study from Duke University in Durham, North Carolina, 68 people with high blood pressure and 32 people with normal blood pressure were given a battery of mental tests. The subjects with high blood pressure showed significant impairments in their short-term memory, and they were slower in processing information.

Eat animals and vegetables for minerals. Be sure to get your fair share of minerals. Boron and zinc may help maintain attention and memory, says James G. Penland, Ph.D., research psychologist with the United States Department of Agriculture's Grand Forks Human Nutrition Research Center in North Dakota. Men fed a diet that supplied 3¼ milligrams of boron a day scored significantly higher on tests of attention, memory and motor performance than when they ate a low boron diet. Good sources of boron are pears, grapes, nuts and tomatoes. In zinc studies, Dr. Penland found that men who consumed less than a third of the daily Recommended Dietary Al-

• •

Spring Wheat

New research at Ball State University in Muncie, Indiana, has been looking into the potential of sprouted wheat—of all things—to retard the aging process. In an experiment, two groups of mice on different diets were doused with cell-damaging x-rays. Half the mice fed a normal diet died within 30 days, but all those fed wheat sprouts continued to live more than six months after the study's end. The researchers suspect sprouts in the diet may also benefit humans.

lowance (RDA), roughly 4 milligrams, performed poorly on memory tests, compared with when they consumed the full RDA of 15 milligrams. For zinc, eat oysters, herring, wheat bran, milk, lean pork and veal.

Double-cross yourself. To unleash your creative juices, "force your brain out of its old grooves," says B. Alexis Castorri, sports therapist and coauthor, with Jane Heller, of *Mental Aerobics: Exercises for a Stronger, Healthier Mind.* To do that, she suggests trying things like rearranging your clothes closet, wearing your watch on the other wrist and brushing your teeth with your nondominant hand. "Creativity means breaking habits and becoming more flexible," she says. Other ways to enhance your creativity: Read a book on an unfamiliar subject, take up a martial art or change your daily newspaper. Or try this mind-stimulating exercise: Spend three minutes dreaming up potential uses for a paper clip.

Go light on the potato salad at lunchtime. According to a Harvard University study, men over age 40 who ate sherbet, which is almost pure carbohydrate, had up to twice the difficulty concentrating and performing mental tasks as a similar group that had eaten turkey. High-protein foods like turkey, chicken, lean beef or fish contain the amino acid tyrosine, which has been linked to clear thinking and alertness.

Graze, don't feast. You know how lethargic you feel after a huge Thanksgiving dinner? Eating a large meal can cause a drop in energy level, because more blood is shunted to the digestive tract (to move out and store all that food) than to your brain. Your mind will function better if you eat smaller meals more often. That plan may also steady your blood sugar and block sleepiness.

Get off the caffeine roller coaster. While coffee keeps you alert, it can also contribute to late-afternoon fogginess. If you tend to hit a mental slump six to eight hours after those morning jolts of French roast, you could be suffering from caffeine withdrawal. It might pay for you to wean yourself from the bean. Best way to quit is slowly. Reduce your intake incrementally by mixing your regular brew with more and more decaffeinated coffee every day.

To bolster your head, apply a pillow. If you want to retain what you've learned during the day, get a sound night's sleep. Studies suggest that dreaming helps to cement memo-

FOG ALERT

Behind the mirrored door of your medicine cabinet is a collection of prescription and nonprescription drugs that can cause drowsiness and make it difficult for you to concentrate. Here are some to be aware of.

- Antihistamines can cause grogginess and impair thought processes.

- High-blood-pressure medications can have mind-fuzzying effects. Two types, beta-blockers and calcium-channel blockers, may also cause fatigue.

- Pain-relievers like ibuprofen cause drowsiness or dizziness in 3 to 15 percent of users. Some sinus/allergy/headache products contain antihistamines that may compound the effect.

- Antinausea agents, such as motion-sickness pills, can cause drowsiness.

- Prescription cough suppressants are often made with codeine, and many over-the-counter cough syrups contain dextromethorphan or diphenhydramine, all of which have potentially sedating effects. Any cough syrup with the title "elixir" contains alcohol, as much as 25 percent, which is more than in a hearty wine. Look for alcohol-free products.

new information. Most of your dreaming is done during a period of sleep called REM (rapid eye movement). Researchers at Israel's Weizmann Institute of Science reported that people won't remember a task they learned very well if they are awakened during REM sleep. But if allowed to sleep undisturbed, test subjects performed newly learned tasks faster and better the next morning.

—*Jeff Stevenson*

Decade-by-Decade Fitness

What we think of as aging may be little more than the result of disuse. Here's a tune-up plan for all ages.

● ● ● ● ● ● ● ● ● ● ● ● ● ● ● ● ● ● ●

AGING MEN, WHEN THEY GET GRUMPY, tend to complain that youth is wasted on the young, but this just isn't so. If anything, youth is wasted on the old, or at least *by* the old. Most of us view our physical youth as some hot sports car that our dad threw us the keys to—we race blithely through life without much more than the occasional refueling, until one day the transmission pops out and some guy in a white smock is shaking his head and telling us we don't pass inspection. It makes more sense to think of a healthy body as a long-term investment that, with the right care, will evolve from trendy roadster to vintage hot rod, still commanding attention whenever it takes to the street.

Of course, you need to put out some effort to keep the machinery of your body active and well-tuned. But with a little bit of work, the payoff can be tremendous. All things considered, any fit, toned man at age 50 can compare his physique, energy and bearing to a 20-year-old's and not find himself wanting. "Two-thirds of what we think of as aging is really disuse," says Walter Bortz, M.D., a 63-year-old marathoner who did some of the pioneering research on how exercise slows the rate of decline in the human body.

Now, if you're like most men, you may have a little trouble fitting marathon training in among work, social life and those endless trips to the hardware store your wife is always forcing you to make. But that's okay, says Dr. Bortz, because his kind of relentless dedication to sports isn't required. Instead, getting in shape should be approached strategically by targeting the areas that need the most attention, depending on your age. When you narrow the focus, you can easily do what's necessary to keep the machinery in working order in three 45-minute workouts a week. (Do check with your doctor before starting any exercise program.) Let's take it by the decade.

THE TWENTIES

"The young have vitality to waste," says Dr. Bortz, a fact that's obvious to anyone who's ever caught an episode of *Club MTV.* But that doesn't mean you have nothing substantial to gain from working out in your twenties. This is a decade for investment, for building up resources that you may be able to draw from later. Of particular importance is bulking up with an aggressive weight-training regimen. There are a number of reasons for this.

First, it'll make you a beautiful specimen. For some men, we need say no more.

Second, at this age the body is still pumping out more than ample amounts of growth hormone, the body chemical that keeps muscles strong. Some research indicates that in young adults, vigorous exercise may actually *increase* the amount of growth hormone you produce. Not so later.

Third, weight training builds bone. Men have the impression that because women start to lose bone mineral earlier than we do (thirties for them, late forties to early fifties for us), osteoporosis isn't a problem for us. That's not so. Men's bones erode, too, which can really hinder mobility further down the pike. The twenties is a time to build up bone density that can then be maintained through later decades, says Gary Hunter, Ph.D., director of the exercise physiology lab at the University of Alabama, Birmingham. It's not that you'll actually prevent future bone loss in this way, "but you'll have a heck of a lot more to spare," says Dr. Hunter.

A final point about the twenties is that it's not too early to start watching your diet, particularly if you're already on the heavy side. Research suggests that men who are overweight in their twenties are almost twice as likely as normal-weight men to add major poundage by their mid-thirties.

The Twenties Workout

Intensity is the key, as a twenty-something body can safely take a high level of physical stress. Pushing yourself hard gains you benefits from aerobic exercise faster at this age, clearing more time for the heavy-duty muscle building you're aiming for.

Monday, Wednesday and Friday

▪ 30 minutes of strength training. Using heavy weights and doing few repetitions will build muscle fastest. After a warm-up, do three sets with enough weight so that you fatigue your muscles after 8 to 12 lifts. Rest about a minute between sets, completing all three sets before moving to the next station. When doing 12 repetitions becomes easy, add enough weight (about 10 percent more) to make it hard again.

At every age, you want a well-rounded weight regimen that hits all the major muscle groups. The basic workout should include:

Bench presses (chest)
Military presses (shoulders)
Lat pulldowns (back)
Leg extensions (quadriceps)
Leg curls (hamstrings)
Biceps curls
Triceps extensions
Crunches or obliques (abdominals)

▪ 15 minutes of aerobic exercise paced at about 80 percent of maximal heart rate. Because your body is still strong and responsive, now's the best time for high-impact exercises.

Ideal sports include football, rugby, soccer, running, baseball, basketball and tennis.

THE THIRTIES

Around the start of your fourth decade, the gradual wearing down that occurs through the rest of life begins oh-so-imperceptibly. Most of the major markers, such as muscle mass, strength, metabolism (the rate at which the body burns fuel) and aerobic capacity, start their dives at the same time, with overall function decreasing at an average rate of about 1 percent a year. But you're still a young man, and the drop-off in your fitness level will not be so noticeable in this decade if you keep active, Dr. Hunter notes.

What the man in his thirties has to watch out for—whether he's active or not—is declining flexibility. Flexibility tapers at about the same rate as other major measures of aging, but the process can start much sooner, in the teens or even earlier, Dr. Hunter says. As a result, while in your thirties, you'll feel the first twinges of creakiness in joints that aren't frequently put through a full range of motion. And nothing makes you feel old faster than the sense that a once-limber body is now less fluid and more constrained.

Keeping yourself flexible doesn't take a lot of effort, and it doesn't mean straining and contorting yourself into a human Gumby. All that's required is that muscles and joints be moved and stretched once in a while. Perhaps because it seems so easy, most men don't set aside the time to make flexibility a priority, says Carol Espel, exercise physiologist and nutritionist at Apex Studios, a New York City health club. "It's the most commonly neglected part of a workout," she observes.

The Thirties Workout

Stick to the basic workout from the twenties, but aim to maintain muscle rather than build it. This lets you shorten your weight workout, dedicate more time to moderate aerobics and, most important, add stretches.

Monday, Wednesday and Friday

- Twenty-five minutes of aerobic exercise at a comfortable pace (70 percent of maximal heart rate).

- Fifteen minutes of strength training, doing two sets using slightly lighter weights and 12 to 15 repetitions, which is ideal for muscle definition.

- Finish with five to ten minutes of stretches. Pay particular attention to back and hamstring muscles. Not only are these extremely important to everyday activity (and in the case of the back, extremely painful when out of whack) but they're also the muscles most likely to be stiffened by sitting at a desk all day.

You can hit both areas with a simple two-step stretch: Lie on your back and draw your knees to your chest. Hold for 30 seconds. This stretches the lower back. Now put both feet flat on the floor, knees bent, and raise your left leg straight up toward the sky. Hold for 30 seconds, then repeat with the right leg. That stretches the hamstrings without putting strain on your back the way you do with similar stretches performed sitting up.

Ideal sports include tennis, racquetball, running, softball and basketball.

THE FORTIES

This is when most men will notice that the thickest part of their torso has headed south to their equator, for a number of age-related reasons. Let us count the ways.

1. The body's fuel-consuming metabolism slows a tad, so it takes longer to burn off the flab. As a result, more of that flab ends up lining your pelt.

2. You lose a certain amount of lean muscle mass (about six pounds for inactive men during their thirties, on average).

3. Having less muscle and a slower metabolism means your body needs fewer calories to stoke its furnace, but you're feeding it the same amount of fuel anyway.

4. Your diet is probably too high in fat, which promptly gets deposited in the long-term storage bulkheads deep in your gut.

These are not insurmountable problems, but they demand that you start getting serious about both proper exercise *and* diet. "All the data says you need both to keep weight off," Espel says.

The most important thing to know about diet is that you can forget about how many calories you eat as long as the mix of those calories is right. The general recommendation on nutrient mix is that you eat about 60 percent carbohydrates, 10 to 15 percent protein and no more than 30 percent fat. Ideally, however, your fat intake should be closer to 20 to 25 percent.

This doesn't have to be awful, taste-wise. A middle-age, 150-pound man who's limiting fat to 25 percent of calories can afford a budget of about 55 grams of fat each day. With that, you could eat a breakfast of cereal with skim milk and a bagel with jam, lunch of a turkey sandwich with lettuce, tomato and Dijon mustard (hold the mayo) plus a yogurt and soft drink, and still be under budget enough to have grilled fish for dinner, with a baked potato and vegetables like green beans and corn. Just go easy on the sour cream and butter you put on those side dishes.

The Forties Workout

Your two basic goals are to subtract fat, which demands that you do aerobic exercise, and add muscle, which requires strength training. The aerobic component becomes even more crucial, because it also boosts cardiovascular fitness, fending off middle-aged concerns like heart attack, stroke and high blood pressure. The one proviso is that you begin paying greater attention to what your body can handle. "People start to injure themselves more at this age," Espel says, usually because they place too much stress on weakening joints. To help accomplish all this, you'll be replacing one day of your standard workout with circuit training. Exercises done on machines are safer; they're sort of like working out with a very careful spotter.

Monday and Friday

- Twenty-five minutes of aerobic exercise at a comfortable pace (60 to 70 percent of maximal heart rate). Avoid getting all your aerobic exercise with high-impact activities like running. If you like to run, do it one day a week, then bike, swim or stair-climb on another day.

- Fifteen minutes of strength training, doing two sets of 12 to 15 repetitions. Consider working with a trainer, if only to help reestablish optimal heaviness levels for these exercises.

- Five to ten minutes of stretches.

Wednesday

- Forty-five minutes of circuit training. Do three circuits, hitting the same weight stations as with the basic workout, but using lighter weights to do 15 to 20 repetitions. Instead of doing all sets of a given station at once and resting in between, do one set, then move quickly to the next exercise. You'll get an aerobic workout that's easy on your joints and exercises all your body's muscles.

Ideal sports include tennis, racquetball, basketball, biking, swimming and fitness walking.

THE FIFTIES

The word here is maintenance. If you've been active so far, it means you've hung on to most of your lean tissue, you have good aerobic capacity, your metabolism is revving nicely and your bones are strong. Now, however, the portion of natural decline that *doesn't* have to do with what Dr. Bortz calls disuse starts to become more obvious. The biggest challenge at this age is not to slack off.

"There's typically a decrease in physical activity with age," says Arthur Weltman, Ph.D., director of the exercise physiology program at the University of Virginia in Charlottesville. "People start to exercise less regularly and less intensely." It's as if many men just give up at this point.

One reason may be that we men think it's necessary to keep up the energy and force of our younger years and find it discouraging that, despite our best efforts, our physical condition deteriorates. But vitality is a relative thing; when you're 50, you shouldn't expect to exercise like a 20-year-old, and, in fact, you don't have to. "Your average 50-year-old has a lower aerobic capacity than your average 20-year-old, so he doesn't have to walk or run as fast to maintain it," Dr. Hunter says. The important thing is that you be fit for *your* age.

The Fifties Workout

The particulars of your program need not vary much from those of your forties, with one exception: It's a good idea to include exercises that strengthen muscles in the back. Bone loss is now kicking in, and research suggests that the loss in the vertebrae can occur twice as rapidly as in other parts of the body.

Monday and Friday

- Twenty minutes of aerobic exercise at a comfortable pace (60 to 70 percent of maximal heart rate). Stick with mostly low-impact exercises like swimming and biking to reduce the risk of injury.

- Twenty minutes of strength training, doing two sets of 12 to 15 repetitions. (Use basic exercises on page 31) Add this back-building exercise to your workout: Lie on your stomach, fingers lightly touching your ears, and slowly lift your head and chest off the floor, keeping your neck straight. Repeat 10 to 20 times.

- Five to ten minutes of stretches.

Wednesday
- Forty-five minutes of circuit training.

Ideal sports include fitness walking, biking, swimming, golf and tennis.

THE SIXTIES

Now's when relatives start worrying that you're going to "strain yourself" or some such thing every time you put on athletic shorts. Don't listen to anybody's thoughts on your capabilities except your doctor's. You can still make fitness gains well into your eighties and nineties, even if you've never exercised a day in your life. In one Tufts University study, people ages 60 to 72 who trained with weights were able to boost the strength of their hamstring muscles by an average of 6.5 percent *per day.* Active men can make gains, too, though because their starting points are higher, gains aren't as dramatic.

If the first goal at this point is not to act like an old man, the second is to be privately very pragmatic about what you can do and achieve. Here's a quick list of practical suggestions.

- Walk, don't run; injury-causing impact stress to the knee will be one-third to one-sixth less. Also, avoid hard surfaces, and wear shoes with good shock absorption.

- Drink lots of water. Older bodies reserve less fluid and may dehydrate faster than younger ones.

- Work out hard enough to be pleasantly tired the next day, but not more.

"There's no evidence that highly fit people gain any tremendous additional edge over moderately active ones," concludes *Men's Health* magazine advisor Bryant Stamford, Ph.D., director of the Health Promotion and Wellness Center at the University of Louisville. "To be active, you don't have to be doing push-ups and wind sprints. The best indication that you're fit enough is feeling good all day."

The Sixties Workout

Don't let anyone talk you out of exercising. You're not an old man unless you view yourself as one.

Monday and Friday

■ Twenty minutes of aerobic exercise at a comfortable pace (60 to 70 percent of maximal heart rate). Your best bet is brisk walking, which provides superior aerobic benefits with minimal risk of injury.

■ Twenty minutes of strength training, doing two sets of basic exercises for 12 to 15 repetitions. If you've never lifted weights, or are returning to them after a long absence, consult your doctor and a trainer before beginning. Do more exercises using machines rather than free weights, which pose a greater risk of injury. Be sure to include a machine that exercises the back.

■ Five to ten minutes of stretches.

Wednesday

■ Thirty to 40 minutes of circuit training.

Ideal sports include golf, fitness walking and swimming. Leisure activities like yardwork can also provide considerable fitness benefits at this age.

—Richard Laliberte

Part 2

HEALTHY EATS

Power Up Your Favorite Foods

Just because they're your favorite foods doesn't mean they can't be good for you. Here are 30 ways to make your favorite foods healthy.

••••••••••••••••••

I<small>T'S SAFE TO SAY THAT</small> the curve representing modern man's meal-preparation time has grown exceedingly short. Where our forefathers were willing to track a caribou for days in order to get a decent steak, now waiting even 20 minutes for a pizza delivery tries our patience.

With time at such a premium, nutrition often suffers. We know that a steady diet of the quick and the packaged jams our bodies with too much fat, salt and cholesterol, but perhaps more important is what these meals aren't doing. Unplanned meals eaten on the run tend to be low in the vitamins that energize us, keep our immune systems strong and charge up our brains. The more time-pressed a man is, the more he needs to be sure his diet is top-notch. "Whether you're a linebacker or a guy in the front office, you've got to put the right diesel in your engine," says Dean Kleinschmidt, head athletic trainer for the New Orleans Saints professional football team.

Usually, it doesn't take any more time to make and eat a nutritious meal than a poor one. Below are 30 no-brainer ways to power up your favorite foods without sacrificing taste—or time. We'll start with a quick explanation of the key ingredients of good nutrition, but if you already know this stuff, skip right ahead to the meals.

Complex carbohydrates: Foods like pastas, breads, cereals, beans, vegetables and fruits are loaded with these. Carbohydrates are a powerful fuel whose calories pump up your energy level, not your waistline.

Fiber: Found in fruits, vegetables, beans and grains, fiber goes through your system like a sponge, absorbing cholesterol and clearing it away. Studies suggest a high-fiber diet also helps prevent colon cancer and may help control blood sugar levels in people with adult-onset diabetes.

Antioxidant vitamins C, E and beta-carotene: Oxidation, the same chemical reaction that causes sliced apples to turn brown, takes place in our bodies and has been linked to cancer, heart disease and the aging process. Antioxidant vitamins, like C, E and beta-carotene, prevent oxygen particles from doing their damage within the body. Top sources of antioxidants are orange juice, sweet red peppers, strawberries and broccoli for vitamin C; wheat germ, olive oil and safflower oil for vitamin E; and carrots, spinach, sweet potatoes and cantaloupe for beta-carotene.

Calcium: Getting enough of this building block of strong teeth and bones can help ward off osteoporosis (men make up 20 percent of all cases), lower blood pressure, prevent kidney stones and reduce LDL (bad) cholesterol. Besides skim milk, fortified orange juice, yogurt, salmon and green leafy vegetables are excellent foods containing calcium.

Potassium: This mineral may lower blood pressure and prevent heart attacks and strokes. Good sources are potatoes, raisins, orange juice and bananas.

B vitamins: Studies show that some of the Bs play important roles in brain function and memory. And B_6 is believed to be important for maintaining a strong immune system. You'll get one or more of the B vitamins from pasta, sunflower seeds, skim milk, chicken breast, bananas, potatoes, clams or chick-peas.

Magnesium: Deficiencies in magnesium may put you at increased risk of heart disease, kidney stones and gallstones. You'll get magnesium from sunflower seeds, wheat germ, spinach and almonds.

Zinc: This mineral, found in wheat germ, oysters and beef, helps your immune system fight off viruses, and it's a key ingredient in the production of healthy sperm.

30 WAYS TO GIVE YOUR FOOD A LIFT

1. Veg up. Energize bottled spaghetti sauce by adding carbohydrate-rich squash, beans, peas, broccoli and onions. Chop the vegetables, zap them in the microwave for 20 or 30 seconds and throw them right in the sauce.

2. Power pasta. Don't like big chunks of vegetables in your sauce? You can get almost double the daily recommended levels of beta-carotene, plus 4.6 grams of fiber, by grating two carrots finely and mixing them in. You won't even know they're there.

3. Galvanize your sauce. Get 500 percent of the Recommended Dietary Allowance (RDA) of zinc, 800 percent of the RDA of vitamin B_{12}, some magnesium and heart-healthy fish oil by adding just six medium oysters to your marinara sauce.

4. Fiber up. Boost dietary fiber in spaghetti 6.4 grams by substituting whole-wheat pasta for the low-fiber white-flour kind.

5. Sub for beef. Raise the fiber and carbohydrate content of your chili—and lower the fat—by cutting the amount of beef you normally use in half and substituting the same amount of red kidney beans. Trim fat in chili even further by substituting ground turkey or chicken breast for the beef.

6. Make vita-sauce. Add vitamin C, beta-carotene and B vitamins to your lasagna by following this quick recipe from *What's Cooking at the Cooper Clinic,* a cookbook from the Dallas fitness center's nutrition department. You can make the entire meal in less than an hour. One helping delivers 3 grams of fiber, 33 grams of carbohydrates, 22 grams of protein and a lot less fat than traditional lasagna.

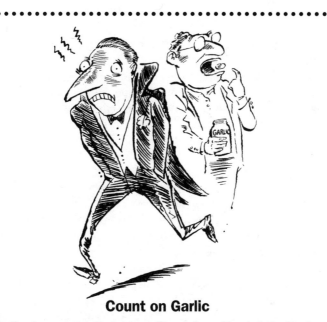

Count on Garlic

Studies have shown that raw garlic can keep blood cholesterol down. Researchers at New York Medical College in Valhalla may have figured out just how much you need to eat each day to make a marked difference. Analyzing data from 28 studies of garlic's effects on serum cholesterol, the researchers concluded that one-half to one clove of garlic a day decreased total cholesterol levels by about 9 percent. An alternative for the bad breath phobic is odor-free garlic tablets, available at health food stores. One pill a day will do it.

Preheat the oven to 375°. Spray the bottom of a 9″ × 12″ casserole dish with no-stick spray. Pour a 28-ounce jar of spaghetti sauce in a bowl and mix in 1 cup water. In another bowl, combine 16 ounces low-fat cottage cheese and ¼ cup part-skim grated mozzarella cheese, ¼ cup fat-free egg substitute, 1 teaspoon garlic powder and ¼ teaspoon pepper. Then, construct your lasagna: Coat the bottom of the dish with sauce, then place a layer of uncooked lasagna noodles on top. Cover the noodles with another layer of sauce, then spoon the cheese mixture over the sauce. Next, add a layer of cooked and drained spinach and/or sliced raw zucchini. Cover the vegetables with a layer of noodles, then sauce, then cheese mixture. Finally, add the remaining sauce, making sure that the noodles are completely covered. Bake uncovered for 50 minutes. Sprinkle some grated mozzarella cheese over the lasagna during the last 15 minutes of baking.

7. Carbo power. Make a high-energy omelette by adding canned, sliced potatoes for more carbohydrate power. Start by mixing two egg whites with two whole eggs to limit the cholesterol. Mix the eggs with sliced mushrooms, sweet red and green bell peppers, onions, the canned potatoes (chopped) and a shot of skim milk, which will add calcium and make the eggs fluffy. You can also take the cholesterol cutting one step further by using fat- and cholesterol-free egg substitutes. You'll find them in the dairy or frozen-food case at the supermarket.

8. Eat some lean. Make a leaner meat stew by substituting chicken for beef. Boost the carbohydrate level by packing in plenty of potatoes, rice or pasta. Here's an easy, high-powered recipe that's delicious.

Get a pound of boneless chicken breasts, 2 cans of low-fat, reduced-salt chicken broth and a 10-ounce package of mixed frozen vegetables. Cut the chicken into chunks. Dump the chicken, vegetables and broth into a pot. Add a chopped clove of garlic, and cook over medium heat about 15 minutes, or until the chicken is done. Then ladle out the chicken and vegetables and place them on a plate. Put 1 cup rice, 1 cup macaroni or pasta shells or 1 large potato (cubed) in the broth. Bring to a boil, then reduce the heat and allow to cook for 10 minutes. Dump the chicken and vegetables back in the pot and simmer for 5 minutes more.

9. Low-fat pizza. Pack your pizza with vitamins by topping the pie with any of the following: broccoli, green bell and sweet red peppers, eggplant, mushrooms, cauliflower and tomato slices. Remember, too, any pizza-improvement project depends as much on what you take off as on what you add on. So before you pile on the vegetables, delete the pepperoni for a savings of 7.6 grams of fat in just two slices. Also, next time you're ordering a pie, ask them to use half the cheese they normally do.

10. Muscular macaroni. Add muscle to macaroni and cheese by sprinkling some crunchy wheat germ on top before baking. One-quarter cup of wheat germ offers 50 percent of the RDA of folate, a B vitamin important to the production of red blood cells, and 40 percent of the RDA for vitamin E. You'll also want to trim the fat by substituting a low-fat sharp cheddar for the regular kind. One brand to try is Kraft Light Naturals Sharp Cheddar Reduced-Fat Cheese. The adventurous eater who wants more fiber and carbohydrates can also add a package of mixed frozen vegetables or a can of white kidney beans or Great Northern beans.

11. Salad days. Make a huge bowl of antioxidant-rich fruit salad and keep it in your refrigerator so you can dip into it all week. In a large bowl, combine the following:

1 pink grapefruit, peeled and sectioned
1 large navel orange, peeled and sectioned
1 sliced mango
1 cup cantaloupe chunks
1 cup honeydew chunks
1 cup strawberry halves
½ cup raspberries or other berries

In a smaller bowl, mix together:

½ cup nonfat vanilla yogurt
2 tablespoons orange juice
1 tablespoon lime juice

Pour the yogurt topping over the fruit and mix well. Spoon onto a plate and sprinkle with sunflower seeds and almond slivers.

12. Be smart at the bar. Make better choices at the salad bar by skipping the iceberg lettuce—it's almost entirely devoid of nutrition—and selecting the darker, leafy vegetables such as romaine, red tip, Boston Bibb and spinach. Top this off with vegetables that have dark yellow, orange and green colors, such as peppers, broccoli and squash. As a rule of thumb, the darker the color of the vegetable, the more nutrients it contains. Also, you can:

- Sprinkle raisins on salads for fiber.

- Top any salad with shredded cabbage. It kicks in vitamin C and fiber.

- Get more copper by adding a few boiled shrimp, sesame seeds, nuts or mushrooms. Copper keeps bones, skin and tendons healthy and may reduce LDL (bad) cholesterol and boost HDL (good) cholesterol.

- Steer clear of the creamy dressings, most of which are loaded with fat. Instead go for vinegar or lemon with just a little olive oil.

13. Power tacos. Power up tacos by increasing the carbohydrates and fiber. Swap canned pinto beans and brown rice for the beef. Here's our favorite recipe.

Coat a large skillet with no-stick spray and heat. Sauté 1 small minced onion and 2 minced cloves of garlic. Then add some chili powder, a pinch of cumin, ¼ cup tomato sauce and ¾ cup water. Bring to a boil, then add a can of drained pinto beans and a cup of quick-cooking brown rice. Cover and simmer for 5 minutes. Remove from heat and let stand another 5 minutes. Spoon into taco shells or tortillas and top with low-fat grated cheddar, hot sauce and shredded lettuce.

14. Brewer's popcorn. Popcorn is one of the healthiest snacks you can eat. A handful of air-popped popcorn has just six calories and is a good source of B vitamins and fiber. Make it even better by sprinkling on a tablespoon of brewer's yeast, available at health food stores. Brewer's yeast adds B vitamins and a good dose of potassium. Also add garlic or chili powder for flavor.

15. Better your burger. Make a better burger by cutting the beef one-to-one with mashed firm tofu in a mixing bowl. (You won't even taste the tofu, and you'll be adding B vitamins and calcium.) Then add chopped onions and whole-wheat bread crumbs for fiber. Mix in some egg white, a little ketchup and dried oregano. Form into patties and cook. Serve it on a whole-wheat roll and top it with romaine lettuce and tomato.

16. Veggie fries. Want some fries to go with the burger? Try zucchini fries. Slice two zucchini into fry-size pieces. Sauté the fries in ½ teaspoon oil in a large pan over medium-high heat

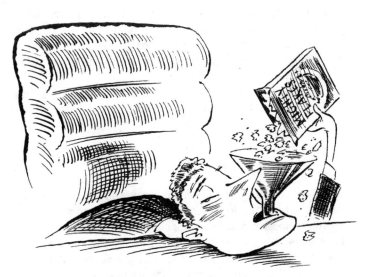

Tank Up with Premium

If your energy peters out by 11:00 A.M. and your stomach grumbles loudly enough for your secretary to hear, you're probably not tanking up with the right fuel at breakfast. Here are some ways to get the extra energy you need to keep your brain and body humming until lunch—without piling on the calories.

- Spread all-fruit preserves on your whole-wheat toast, paired with a bowl of whole-grain cereal.
- Eat low-fat dairy foods: Have skim milk on your cereal or some yogurt or low-fat cottage cheese with fruit.
- If you crave meat in the morning, fry up some Canadian bacon. It is lower in fat than regular bacon or sausage, making it a good choice for an occasional treat.

until lightly browned. Sprinkle with basil. Or if you like things hot, sprinkle with Cajun spices.

17. Surf barbecue. Make a better barbecue with fish in place of meat. Not only is fish a good source of protein, it also contains omega-3 fatty acids, a good-for-you type of fat that may ward off heart disease. Fish also contains magnesium, B vitamins and potassium. The best fish for grilling: tuna, salmon, red snapper, halibut, bluefish and swordfish.

18. Grill lean. Grill leaner by cooking a turkey. Buy a thick, palm-size slab of turkey tenderloin, which is the leanest cut on the bird. Marinate it in a bowl of bottled low-fat Italian salad dressing for ten minutes. Toss it on the grill over high heat to brown both sides, about three minutes a side. Heat up an individual round pizza shell in a toaster oven for two minutes. Then wrap the shell around your turkey filet, sandwich-like, and top with chunky salsa.

19. Pie pleasure. Get all the pleasure of apple pie with apple crisp instead. You gain cholesterol-lowering oats and you

· ·

HEALTH FOOD IMPOSTORS

Just because you find it at health food stores, and ruddy-faced outdoors types eat it, that doesn't mean it should be on *your* plate. Look beyond appearances and check out what's inside.

1. Granola. The majority of granolas on the market are loaded with fat, as much as 27 grams in a single serving. And that's without milk. "Traditional granolas are high in coconut oil, a saturated fat, and that's the worst kind for you," says Martin Yadrick, R.D., a nutritionist and spokesman for the American Dietetic Association. There are low-fat varieties, but read the label before you indulge. Rule of thumb: If it has more than 2 grams of fat per serving, pass it by.

2. Bran muffins. Ever notice how some bran muffins leave your napkin and your hands greasy? That's from all the oil inside. A typical small bran muffin contains 4 grams of fat, and some large ones may have as much as 12 grams and 900 calories. Opting for a bagel gets you down to 1.4 grams of fat and 160 calories.

· ·

lose almost all the fat. Here's an easy recipe to try.

Peel, core and slice eight medium-size apples and place them in an oven-proof bowl coated with no-stick spray. In a separate bowl, mix together ½ cup raisins, 2 tablespoons lemon juice, ¾ cup whole-wheat flour and 1¼ cups oats. Drizzle with ½ cup apple juice, ⅓ cup honey or brown sugar and 2 tablespoons canola oil. Add 1 teaspoon cinnamon. Sprinkle this mixture over the apples and bake at 350° for about 30 to 40 minutes, or until the apples are tender. Serve with a topping of vanilla frozen yogurt.

60-Second Power Boosters

Here are 11 more quick techniques for taking your meals to another level, nutrition-wise.

20. Strong bones. Nearly double your intake of calcium and protein from a glass of milk, without adding fat. Mix two tablespoons of nonfat dry milk in an eight-ounce glass of cold skim milk. It'll make the skim milk thicker, too.

3. Apple juice. Apples are a terrific source of vitamin C and fiber. But apple juice is little more than sugar water. You're better off with a glass of cranberry juice, which is loaded with vitamin C.

4. Frozen yogurt. Some brands of frozen yogurt contain up to seven grams of fat per serving. Read the label, and don't bring home any brand with more than three grams of fat per serving. Try Colombo's nonfat yogurt, I Can't Believe It's Yogurt! nonfat, and TCBY's nonfat flavors.

5. Carob. Carob candy won't save you from the sins of chocolate. Both contain virtually the same amount of fat, and at least chocolate doesn't taste like rabbit pellets.

6. Trail mix. It's fine to munch on nuts, seeds and dried fruit for energy during a ten-mile hike, but don't eat handfuls of the stuff at home. The seeds and nuts are loaded with fat, and the dried fruit contains lots of calories. Fresh fruit or pretzels are better snacks.

21. Bean power. Power-pack prepared soups by adding a can of beans or crushed tomatoes to the simmering pot. Increase fiber by adding barley to vegetable soups.

22. Spreadables. Try fruit spreads on your toast instead of butter. Apple butter spread, for example, offers 38 milligrams of potassium per tablespoon and virtually no fat.

23. Vita-ice. Substitute frozen melon balls for ice cubes in fruit drinks. A half-cup of honeydew melon has 230 milligrams of potassium and 20 milligrams of vitamin C.

24. Skim stew. Trim the fat off stews and soups by cooking them a day early and chilling them overnight. In the morning, skim off the hardened fat.

25. Skin game. Eat fruits and vegetables with their skins and peels intact for more fiber. For the same reason, eat the membranes that cling to oranges and grapefruit when you peel them.

26. Bran breasts. Bread chicken breasts with bran cereal before baking them to load some fiber into the meal.

27. Beta-punch. Add a handful of fresh parsley to stews, soups and sauces for a punch of beta-carotene.

28. Freezer fiber. Keep a bag of frozen corn in your freezer and use it to add fiber and carbohydrates to any meal. Toss one-half cup into whatever's cooking to add 17 grams of carbohydrate and 1.6 grams of dietary fiber.

29. Fling grits. Fling a handful of soy grits—available in health food stores—into chili and stews. Soy adds B vitamins, calcium and zinc. And you'll hardly know it's there.

30. Skim power. Raise calcium levels by sprinkling skim-milk powder into mashed potatoes, gravies and sauces.

—Jeffrey Csatari

Lose Fat, Gain Muscle

Fat exacts a heavy tax on your body. But this is one taxing load you can do something about. It's time to ease your personal fats burden.

• • • • • • • • • • • • • • • • • • • •

IN AN ONGOING EFFORT TO ENSURE domestic tranquillity, recent administrations have treated us to a stream of images designed to show off our presidents' virility. For four years, George Bush jogged, raced around in boats, played golf—anything to prove his fitness and lay aside fears that Dan Quayle might suddenly become president. Before that, Ronald Reagan chopped wood in his backyard, displaying his own vim and vigor and trying to quell fears that one day George Bush might become president.

The current talismans of presidential fitness are the constant photos of Bill Clinton running through the streets of Washington with a dozen panting G-men and a couple of visiting celebrities in tow. But the almost daily images of the 205-pound Clinton in his sweat-soaked jogging attire make one wonder—if this guy is so into exercise, how come he's still so heavy? Why do his joint press conferences with Boris Yeltsin look more like Sumo wrestling matches than summit meetings? Why can't Bill Clinton lose that weight?

There's a lesson to be learned here, and it's basically this: You can exercise until you wear holes in the soles of your cross-trainers, but unless you're smart about what you eat, you won't get that belly under control. And just because you're the president, that doesn't mean you know any more about nutrition than the average school board electee. Clinton's diet is like most Americans': heavy on the meat and always followed by dessert. He also likes to nosh at midnight. One presidential late-night snack reportedly consisted of cocktail shrimp, pastries, mango sorbet and French bread dripping with olive oil.

Not so healthy, but wait—can't you just work out a little harder to burn off those extra calories? Kind of like spending your way out of a recession? Not really. This is a supply-side issue. Let's say, for example, you run three miles at a clip of about eight minutes each—approximately President Clinton's pace on an average weekday. Then you stop at McDonald's and order a Big Mac. What you've just done is burn off 384 calories, then immediately pile 500 back on.

EAT MORE, NOT LESS

Everybody knows that this is not good. In order to lose weight, you need to burn off more calories than you take in. So one might logically think, if I eat less food, I'll reduce the number of calories I'm taking in, and in no time I'll be fitting into those size 32 jeans I wore to peace marches at Oxford in 1968. Sorry, Bubba—not even if you inhale. In fact, strict diets are for chumps. The best way for any man to lose weight is to eat *more,* not less. As long as you eat more of the right things.

That's because your body is a highly evolved masterpiece adept at keeping itself alive even during times of starvation. And when you go on a diet, that's exactly what's happening—you're starving yourself. According to nutrition experts, diets don't work because when you deprive your body of food, your metabolic rate—the speed with which you burn calories—actually *drops* as the body tries to fight off what it thinks is starvation. So instead of using up your extra fat, your body clings to your love handles, unwilling to let them go lest the famine continue.

So the key is not to eat less, but to eat less of the foods that make you fat and more of the foods that keep your metabolism revving. For example, let's say you and the president have diets that are about 40 percent fat—that's the average for Americans. Every gram of fat you eat comes jam-packed with nine weighty calories. By contrast, protein and carbohydrates have only four calories per gram. That means that for every gram of fat you cut out of your daily diet, you can add twice as many grams of carbohydrates and still be eating fewer calories. More food, fewer calories. Get it?

But replacing fat with carbohydrates works for another reason. Your body loves to convert dietary fat into body fat, because the transformation takes almost no energy. On the other hand, your body burns up almost ten times as many calories converting protein or carbohydrates into body fat. So it instead uses all the grains, fruits and vegetables for immediate energy and waits for that evening slice of cheesecake to make its way into your belly. A moment on the lips, a lifetime on the hips, as they say.

LESS FAT, MORE PLEASURE

The question remains, how does one cut down on fat without destroying the pleasure of eating? We wouldn't put the commander-in-chief on a diet of grapefruit, tofu and water, and we wouldn't ask you to go on one, either. You don't need to deprive yourself to eat healthy, says Martin Yadrick, R.D., a nutritionist and spokesman for the American Dietetic Association. For example, let's say you're a certain leader of a certain Free World with an overachieving wife and a bizarre genetic resistance to male pattern baldness. Or you're just some guy. Either way, here are the easy-to-follow rules.

1. Remember that many foods are naturally low in fat and jam-packed with the nutrients and fiber you need to keep you running. Not that you should stuff yourself, but within reason you can pretty much eat all you want of the following foods.

- Grains, like pasta, bread, rice, oats, barley and cereals, as long as they haven't been weighted down with fat and sugar. (Sorry, beer doesn't count as a barley product.)

- Beans and legumes, such as kidney beans, peas, black beans, lentils, pinto beans and so on.

• •

Just Desserts

If you think you're eating right by choosing a salad or low-fat chicken sandwich for lunch, take a closer look at what you're eating for dinner. Research has found that people who believe they're eating a low-fat meal tend to reward themselves with fatty foods afterward. Nondieting volunteers who were told they were getting low-fat lunches took in more fat than usual from the rest of their meals according to one study.

SLIMMING DOWN THE BIG ENCHILADA

You *can* cut fat without cutting out your favorite foods.

Just to prove how pain-free fighting fat can be, we made a few tasteful substitutions in one of Bill Clinton's favorite dishes—chicken enchiladas. He likes them the way they're prepared at one of his Arkansas haunts, Trio's: filled with cheese and topped with a gooey cream sauce.

A traditional enchilada recipe calls for dipping the tortillas briefly into hot fat, then dipping them into the sauce and wrapping the chicken, onions and cheese with them. They are then placed in a well-oiled pan, covered with more sauce and baked for ten minutes. They're served topped with sour cream. Sounds delicious, until you look at the stats: Two enchiladas provide you with 925 calories, 57 percent of which come from fat, and 142 milligrams cholesterol.

Now take the simple substitutions we offer and try this: Warm the tortillas in an oven, without oil, and spray the baking pan with no-stick spray. For the sauce, sauté the onions and garlic in water or stock instead of oil. The results: 590 calories, 30 percent fat and 95 milligrams cholesterol.

- All fruits.

- Vegetables like potatoes, carrots, asparagus, peppers, sweet potatoes and even that bane of the Bush kitchen, broccoli.

2. Cows are fat factories, so be moderate in your consumption of whole-milk dairy products. Look for skim milk and low-fat versions of yogurt, cheese and sour cream. If you're drinking whole milk now, make the switch to skim gradually, starting with 2 percent milk and working your way down over a month or so. By the time you're done, skim will be just as satisfying as whole milk used to be.

3. When it comes to meat, most of us eat too much. Hardliners suggest you cut out meat altogether, but if you can't live without an occasional roast beef sandwich, at least cut down

Old Recipe	New Recipe
1 whole chicken breast, poached	Same
¾ pound Monterey Jack cheese	¾ pound Kraft Monterey Jack Lite
1 onion, chopped	Same
8 flour tortillas	8 corn tortillas
2 tablespoons vegetable oil	No-stick pan spray
1 cup sour cream	1 cup fat-free sour cream

Tomatillo sauce	Our sauce
1 onion, minced	Same ingredients, but substitute water or stock for oil
2 cloves garlic, minced	
2 tablespoons vegetable oil	1½ cups fresh tomatillos
1 can chopped green chilies	
1 chopped jalapeño	
½ teaspoon sugar	
salt to taste	

on your consumption as much as possible. Six ounces a day is the most you want, says Yadrick, and even that is pushing it, so don't think that if you have rice and beans tonight you can have a huge porterhouse this weekend. A typical serving of meat should be about the size of a deck of cards.

Of course, not all meat dishes are created equal. Here are some guidelines.

- A painless way to cut down on meat is to look for dishes where meat is an ingredient, not the centerpiece, of the meal. Examples include stir-fries, chili, spaghetti with meat sauce or stews.

- Poultry is generally lower in fat than red meat, but you have to know the bird. Meat from the breast is less fatty than dark meat from the legs or wings, and removing the skin will cut a considerable amount of fat. Avoid fried chicken like the plague.

- When eating fish, steamed or broiled is your best bet. As for shellfish, choose those that don't swim, such as clams, mussels, scallops and oysters. They are the vegetarians of the sea, and as a result they are lower in fat than lobster, shrimp or crab.

4. Beware of oils of all kinds. That includes oil-containing products, such as margarine and most salad dressings. Remember that all oils are liquid fat, even olive oil, safflower oil and canola oil. Look out for these hidden sources of oil: avocados, olives, nuts and seeds.

5. If you're taking the easy way out and buying prepackaged foods, look for low-fat products like Healthy Choice frozen meals, Health Valley chili (and many other Health Valley products), Kraft Free nonfat mayonnaise and salad dressings, Guiltless Gourmet tortilla chips, Quaker Oats oatmeal, Nabisco fat-free crackers, Fleischmann's Egg Beaters, Pritikin soups, Light 'N Lively Free nonfat sour cream, Häagen-Dazs frozen yogurt bars and Entenmann's fat-free desserts.

Remember, your weight is primarily influenced by how much fat you eat, not how many miles you run. But with a few modest changes in your choice of fuel, you could be as fit and trim as Al Gore. So next time you jog all sweaty into a fast-food joint, remember this key phrase: "It's the fat, stupid."

—Stephen Perrine

E-Male Message

Even if you've never taken vitamins before . . . even if you're in no special hurry to start . . . this is one you'd better think twice about.

• • • • • • • • • • • • • • • • • • •

WALK INTO ANY HEALTH-AND-NUTRITION OUTLET and you'll be overwhelmed by the array of pills and lotions and ground-up herbs that do . . . well, who knows what? Grow hair? End flatulence? Get Naomi Campbell to do your bidding? It's so confusing, no wonder so many of us shy away from taking vitamins and supplements.

But what if we told you that there among the dillweed water and tincture of goat marrow was a single capsule that, taken every day, could protect you from heart disease and cancer, preserve your eyesight, shore up your muscles and maybe boost your brain power in the bargain?

Let's cut to the chase: That miracle pill is plain old vitamin E, and the latest research on this humble nutrient is nothing short of astounding.

You may already have heard about the benefits of antioxidants, which include vitamins C and E and beta-carotene. This trio of nutrients targets *free radicals,* rogue molecules that fasten on to other molecules and cause a heap of damage. Free radicals in the air are what cause iron to rust and meat to turn brown. In the body, they cause skin to wrinkle and blood vessels to clog, and, over time, they can weaken the immune system, leading to a broad array of diseases.

Essentially, free radicals are like stag gentlemen at a couples-only party. All they want to do is hook up with another molecule, and they don't care what kind of trouble they cause when they do. Antioxidants are like bouncers—they take the free radicals by the arm and lead them out of the dance hall, preventing them from making mischief. And researchers are discovering that, because vitamin E works so well at eliminating free radicals just about anywhere—in blood vessels, muscles, the lens of the eye—it is right at the front of the antioxidant pack.

All right, you might say, I'm a happy, healthy guy—what is vitamin E going to do for me? According to the latest research, a lot.

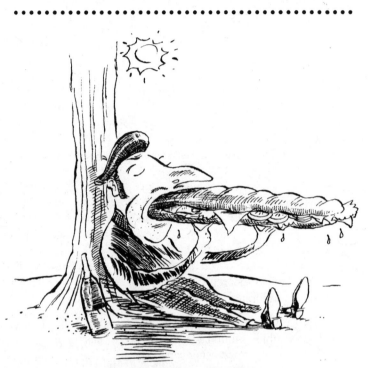

You Are When You Eat

It may not only be what you eat, but also when you eat that makes a difference to your health. Take the French, for example: They devour piles of pâté, slabs of Camembert and some of the richest pastries known to man, and still they're far less likely to die of heart disease than Americans are. To get to the bottom of the matter, researchers at Boston University School of Medicine compared the eating patterns of middle-class Parisians with those of their American counterparts. They observed that the French took their main meal at midday, didn't snack for the next five hours and then ate a light supper, while Americans consumed most of their calories late in the day, including a heavy supper. Eating the bulk of daily calories early may be a key to a healthy heart, since it gives the body more waking hours to burn off all that food.

Block heart disease. Last year, a group from the Harvard School of Public Health looked at the history of vitamin use among almost 40,000 male health professionals in the 40 to 75 age bracket. They found that those who took vitamin E supplements of at least 100 international units (IU) a day for two or more years had a 37 percent lower risk of heart disease than those who did not. The vitamin appears to neutralize free radicals in the artery wall that would otherwise cause the buildup of artery-clogging plaque, according to study leader Eric Rimm, Sc.D.

Lower cancer risk. Researchers speculate that E may prevent free radicals from causing tumor-promoting damage to DNA, the molecule that directs how cells reproduce, or that it may stimulate an immune-system attack on early-stage tumor cells.

- A National Cancer Institute study reported that those who took vitamin E supplements halved their risk of mouth and pharynx cancer.

- In a dietary analysis of 800 nonsmokers, vitamin E supplements were linked with a 45 percent lower risk of lung cancer (although it doesn't appear to help if you insist on smoking).

- A study comparing colorectal cancer patients to healthy subjects found a link between increasing blood levels of E and decreasing cancer risk.

Reduce muscle damage from exercise. A U.S. Department of Agriculture (USDA) nutrition study found that 800 IU of vitamin E a day protected formerly sedentary men— some in their twenties, the rest between ages 55 and 74—from muscle damage following a punishing workout on a treadmill. That's important news for weekend athletes, because free radicals can prey on muscle cells after an intense workout, leaving you sore.

Boost immunity. Vitamin E may block free radicals and other cell chemicals from shutting down immune-cell production and activity. In another USDA study, healthy men and women took 400 IU of vitamin E every day for six months. In those under age 30, one measure of their immune system's function soared 58 percent. In those over 65, immune function nearly doubled.

Prevent cataract formation. Doctors at the Johns Hopkins Medical Institutions evaluated the antioxidant intake of 660 people over age 40 and found that the group with the lowest blood levels of vitamin E had twice the risk of developing cataracts deep within the lens. Why? Free radicals again. It's believed they cause age-related cataracts by attacking certain proteins in the lens of the eye.

Benefit people with diabetes. People with non-insulin-dependent diabetes tend to have lower blood levels of vitamin E and more wayward free radicals as well, which may contribute to poor blood sugar control. But in one study, diabetics who took 900 IU of vitamin E a day for four months showed signs of improved insulin activity and faster glucose removal from the blood.

Delay or prevent Alzheimer's disease. Vitamin E may protect nerve cells from a toxic protein known to accumulate in the damaged brain tissue of people with Alzheimer's disease. Very preliminary lab tests at the Salk Institute for Biological Studies in San Diego indicate that vitamin E prevents the protein from attacking cultures of the affected nerve cells.

Keep in mind that the studies outlined above have established only a link, not a definitive cause-and-effect relationship, between vitamin E and good health. Still, in the minds of many researchers, there's plenty of evidence to justify taking a daily pill. "I recommend men considering vitamin E supplementation of 100 to 400 IU a day," says Jeffrey Blumberg, Ph.D., associate director/senior scientist and chief of the antioxidants research

• •

Take My Wife's Diet, Please

Guys planning to revamp their diets will have a better shot at success if they first get the women in their lives to start eating better. A survey of nearly 400 couples found that husbands of wives on low-fat diets received only 33 percent of their calories from fat, compared with 37 percent of calories from fat for men married to women not on low-fat diets. Percentage of men who suggested their wives go on a diet and spent the next two weeks sleeping on the couch? Don't ask.

laboratory at the U.S. Department of Agriculture Human Nutrition Research Center on Aging at Tufts Universtiy in Medford, Massachusetts. While that's less than the amounts taken in some of the studies above, Dr. Blumberg says his recommended dosages will deliver the same benefits when taken over a long period. In fact, he warns against going out and swallowing whole bottles of E. Amounts in excess of 1,200 IU a day won't give any added benefit—and high doses can cause problems if you're on blood-thinning medications such as Warfarin. Looking for dietary sources of the nutrient? Good choices include fortified cereals (up to 30 IU per serving), sunflower seeds (27 IU per quarter cup) and sweet potatoes (8 IU per one medium, baked).

—*Carol Ann Shaheen*

Best and Worst Midnight Snacks

Late late chow can really blow up your waistline. Here's how to enjoy the late night mirth without adding to your personal girth.

• • • • • • • • • • • • • • • • • •

IT'S 11:30, AND WITHOUT THINKING, I've clicked the remote to NBC. Which is bad news. Because as the technicolor curtains part and Jay's head pops up on the screen, I can only think of one thing: those old Doritos commercials. The saliva flows, the cabinets call, and next thing, I've blown an entire day of reasonably disciplined eating in a single binge. Then I'm in bed, either restless with indigestion or wrestling with another nightmare: Instead of summoning delta waves, I'm being chased by Delta Burke wielding a spiced beef stick.

But, while chips and salami aren't the best of snacks, that doesn't mean a man must be forced to ignore the rumblings of his stomach in the midnight hour. We've consulted the experts and come up with some of the best foods to satisfy you, foods that won't cut into your sleep or leave you stuffed. First, though, the six principles of nighttime eating:

1. Don't have a cow. Meats and other high-protein foods are a mistake before bed. Protein supplies the brain with the amino acid tyrosine, which boosts alertness. "This is the last thing you want when you're trying to sleep," says Judith Wurtman, Ph.D., nutrition researcher in the Department of Brain and Cognitive Science at the Massachusetts Institute of Technology in Cambridge. Foods high in protein also tend to be high in fat, which digests slowly and makes sleep more fitful. So think twice before grabbing for that cold roast beef, not to mention the cheddar, fontina or Swiss cheese.

2. Break bread before bed. Your body starts processing carbohydrates—such as rice, potatoes and bread—immediately. Furthermore, they help speed tryptophan, a sleep-inducing amino acid, to the brain. "Diets that don't contain enough carbohydrates usually turn people into insomniacs," says Dr. Wurtman.

3. Watch for hidden caffeine. Most of us know not to down five cups of coffee before sleeping, but insidious caffeine sources abound. An 8-ounce cup of tea and a 12-ounce can of cola both contain around 35 milligrams of caffeine, about equal to a 4-ounce cup of instant coffee. Many drugstore decongestants and nonprescription painkillers also include caffeine. Two tablets of regular-strength Anacin, for example, have 64 milligrams. Beware of chocolate as well; if you're craving it, try some hot chocolate, which has only 4 milligrams of caffeine.

4. Doff the nightcap. Booze may help you fall asleep faster, but alcohol disrupts your rest by reducing deep sleep and dream sleep—the phases of sleep that leave you refreshed.

5. Avoid the heat in the night. Spicy foods can generate a lot of stomach acid; when you're lying down, the acid can easily back up into the lower esophagus and cause heartburn—and nightmares. "You may feel as though you're being stabbed with an ice pick, when in fact it's just the pepperoni you ate," says Dr. Wurtman. Either that, or you've seen *Basic Instinct* too many times.

6. Punishment for gluttons. Finally, if you're an incorrigible midnight gourmand, here's an incentive to hold the line against overindulging. Many experts believe that food eaten at night has more of a chance of being stored as body fat than the same food eaten in the daytime. James O. Hill, Ph.D., an obesity researcher at the University of Colorado's Center for Human Nutrition in Denver, explains that this is likely because there are fewer bodily functions occurring while you sleep that require energy. The net result: "More of the food you're eating is going into storage," he says.

THE PICK OF THE LOT

Here are the midnight snacks that should top your list.

English muffin pizza. Start by cracking open an English muffin, then spoon on tomato sauce and sprinkle it with a couple of tablespoons of grated low-fat mozzarella. (You can add a pinch of oregano if you want to get fancy.) Throw your concoction in the toaster oven or run it under the broiler for a few minutes. All told, this snack is under 400 calories, with less than ten grams of fat. That's less than half the fat in two slices of pepperoni pizza from Pizza Hut.

Another option is to check out the frozen-food section of your supermarket. In recent years, someone's figured out how to make low-fat versions of pizza that still taste pretty good. We like Weight Watchers pepperoni pizza and Stouffer's Lean Cuisine French bread pizzas. Neither brand contains more than 350 calories or 11 grams of fat.

Turkey breast sandwich. Talk about sandwiches and the mind turns to Dagwood, a man well-attuned to his instincts, though, as a consequence, perhaps not a pillar of self-control. The fact is, a sandwich can be a sensible snack. Two ounces of turkey breast is nearly 13 times less fattening than the same amount of beef salami. Other good sandwich fillers include lean roast beef, grilled chicken cutlet or any kind of non-

• •

Just the Flax, Man

If you switched from white bread to whole wheat to get more fiber, there may be reason to switch again. In one study, eating flaxseed bread lowered cholesterol levels nearly twice as much as eating whole-wheat bread. According to the researchers, several major bread bakers are planning to introduce flaxseed bread to supermarkets soon.

breaded fish. In the shrink-wrapped deli category, Healthy Choice makes a good thin-sliced cooked ham (about half a gram of fat per three slices) and turkey breast (about one gram of fat per three slices).

As a reward for going light on the filling, treat yourself to a good, hearty bread such as whole grain or pita or French bread—any kind is high in carbohydrates and low in fat. But go easy on the toppings, which can blow your whole day's fat budget in a single swipe. Best bets: reduced-calorie or fat-free mayonnaise, low-fat or fat-free salad dressing, and as much lettuce, tomatoes and mushrooms as you want.

Wait, you say you need cheese, too? Okay, but choose low-fat versions and keep the portions light. Borden makes excellent low-fat American, cheddar, mozzarella and Swiss cheeses, all with 35 calories and two grams of fat per slice.

Sundae. If you're in the mood for ice cream, instead go for nonfat frozen yogurt or sherbet for ten grams of fat savings over premium ice cream. Top it with all the fruit you want, sliced bananas, blackberries or strawberries, but hold off on the nuts. Finally, pour on some Estee ChocoSyp, a chocolate syrup with no fat and only 20 calories per tablespoon. Frozen yogurts we like include Häagen-Dazs low-fat, TCBY nonfat flavors and Yoplait low-fat vanilla orange cremes (popsicles). American Glace also makes a good nonfat frozen dessert. Got to have ice cream? Try one of the new nonfat kinds, such as Sealtest, which is delicious.

Cereal. Breakfast cereal makes one of the best midnight snacks. Cornflakes are only 100 calories per cup and have no fat. Most any of the other cereals will do just as well, and if you're man enough to use skim milk, you almost can't go wrong. For those who love granola, check out Kellogg's Low-Fat Granola, which has whole oats and wheat, but no cholesterol and less than half the fat (two grams) of the other granolas.

Cheese-flavored popcorn. Start with air-popped popcorn and add a shake of grated Parmesan or Romano cheese—total fat content: 2.1 grams. Other flavorings to experiment with include chopped dates, raisins or cinnamon. Among commercial varieties, check out Boston's Lite Gourmet Popcorn (three grams of fat) or Weight Watchers White Cheddar Cheese Popcorn (four grams of fat).

Pretzels. These offer a great low-fat, low-sodium alterna-

tive to chips. Wege markets an excellent variety made from natural sourdough bread (less than a gram of fat per serving). But,
if you're an avowed chip man, try the no-oil baked tortilla chip
from Guiltless Gourmet, which has 1.5 grams of fat per serving.
The company also makes an excellent barbecue/pinto bean dip.

Baked goods. Snackwell's Fat Free Devil's Food Cookie
Cakes are a fine example of the trend to low-fat and nonfat
desserts. More good baked goods: Entenmann's Fat-Free
Chocolate Crunch Cake and Weight Watchers Double Fudge
Cake (frozen).

Low-fat cookies. We like Entenmann's oatmeal raisin
cookies. At only 80 calories for every 2, with no fat, these are a
fine choice for cookie-munchers. Another kind we like is R. W.
Frookies apple spice cookies—also with no fat. Or steal your
kid's animal crackers; 13 of them can have fewer than two
grams of fat. Other good grocery buys include Sunshine
Golden Fruit Raisin Biscuits and Pepperidge Farm Wholesome
Choice carrot walnut cookies.

Snack bars. Try the Sunsweet California prune and almond Bar. More nutritious than an Almond Joy any night, this
fruit and nut bar is lightly coated with chocolate, so there's
only a moderate amount of fat (six grams). Other high-
carbohydrate, low-fat "sports bars" are also great at night.
Some of these take a little getting used to, but we liked Power-
Bar's Wild Berry, the citrus-flavored Edgebar and the oat-
bran-flavored Exceed sports bar. Most cost $1.69. For those
craving peanut butter, which is normally loaded with fat, Fi-
Bar makes a vanilla peanut butter crunch snack bar with four
grams of fat—one-fourth of what you'd get in two tablespoons
of peanut butter.

Licorice. Twizzlers and other licorice-type candies are
good nonfat alternatives to candy bars. Other good ways to satisfy your craving for sweets without getting any fat: hard candies, gummy bears, jelly beans.

Fruit with cottage cheese. One cup of blackberries contains loads of fiber and half the daily requirement of vitamin C,
plus they're low in calories, sodium, cholesterol and fat. Combine them with low-fat cottage cheese, and you have a snack
under 160 calories. Sliced pears, apples or apricots are equally
good as toppings, as are dried fruits.

—David Zinczenko

Part 3

MEN AT EASE

Blow Off Stress

They're out there . . . job worries, trouble at home, death and taxes. But you can fight back. Here's how to get a handle on the ten worst male stressors.

• • • • • • • • • • • • • • • •

BACK IN THE OLD DAYS, a guy could see stress coming. Stress looked exactly like Indians on the horizon, Germans in Poland, a private eye with a camera at the motel room door. Until lately, most men knew stress because stress came in a familiar package. It was big and warlike and required a deep breath, a Hail Mary and some variation on the mantra "Suck it up."

No longer. Stress in the '90s comes in much fuzzier, much more free-form components, according to a variety of experts who specialize in men's issues. Stressors, as the experts call these anxiety factors, are now much harder to recognize. Suddenly, there are new rules for everything and new, ballpark-size doubts. What makes a man a success? Fulfilled? A good provider? A good father? A stand-up colleague? You know, a man.

Anyone?

"Ambiguity is killing us," says Steven Berglas, Ph.D., director of the Executive Stress Clinic in Boston. We don't even know how to think about these new problems, let alone come up with answers. Not long ago, the rules of life's game for men were eloquent in their simplicity—play fair, don't hit, be nice to girls, work hard, don't cry, pray in private. That game's over. Now it's a new game. Now, writes humorist Garrison Keillor, author of *The Book of Guys*, "What you find is terrible gender anxiety, guys trying to be Mr. Right, the man who can bake the cherry pie, go shoot skeet, come back, toss a salad, converse easily about intimate matters, cry if need be, laugh, hug, be vulnerable, perform passionately that night and the next day go off and lift them bales onto that barge and tote it. Being perfect is a terrible way to spend your life, and guys are not equipped for it anyway"—and, a reasonable man might add, even if we were equipped for it, we've already seen what trying to "have it all" has done for women who aspire to perfection.

But forget trying to have it all. These days, just showing up for life as a guy can be complex and difficult. Given the constant, ceaseless, often contradictory, often meaningless demands for male adaptation, a man could be King of Bliss and still find himself twisted into a full-stress knot.

The best way to untangle that knot, say the experts, is to attack it one strand at a time. Accordingly, here's our top-ten list from hell, the major stress-makers in a modern man's life.

TRUE ANXIETY ONE: IT COULD BE YOU NEXT

We'll start, randomly, with the rubble and ruin that decorate a once-peaceful corner of a man's world—work, that haven of security and camaraderie, where all the rules were in the job description, where a man always knew where he stood, where overtime paid off, where everybody complained about their wives but didn't mean it, and where venerable old-timers worked shoulder-to-shoulder with newcomers until they retired.

No more. One of the biggest growth industries in the Western world right now is in job and unemployment counseling. Never before have so many pink slips been given to so many by so few with so little notice. Titanic corporations—once the Gibraltars of job security—are announcing layoffs of tens of thousands of workers. Huge disruptions in the labor market are a daily fact of life. American men aged 35 to 54 are 25 percent more likely in the '90s to suffer permanent layoff or job loss than in the previous decade, according to a recent study by Harvard University's James Medoff, Ph.D.

The looming possibility of unemployment really hits us where we live, since we men, far more than women, define ourselves by the jobs we hold. "Nothing is more important to a man's pride, self-respect, status and manhood than work," argues Willard Gaylin, M.D., professor of psychiatry at Columbia University, in his book *The Male Ego.*

So when the man next door—say, a 25-year middle-management veteran of NYNEX or AT&T—suddenly shows up at the front door selling Mary Kay for men, it terrifies us, because we know we could be next. In the 1990s, nobody's job is safe. What that means is that just going to work is a daily dip in an icy reality bath. The pleasure we take in our jobs serves only to remind us how quickly and easily that pleasure can be taken away, and how suddenly we can be forced back out into a world of random misfortune.

TRUE ANXIETY TWO: YOU'RE NOT AS GOOD AS YOUR OLD MAN

All of us are snail darters and spotted owls in a world where Rush Limbaugh is environmental czar. As male bread-winners, we are a threatened, if not endangered, species. Real wages have declined severely for men over the last two decades, and living paycheck to paycheck is increasingly the norm. In this scenario, buying your first home (or more specifically, coming up with a chunk of money for a down payment) is an almost heroic accomplishment—and one that fewer and fewer of us will ever experience. Financial planners advise young breadwinners to start saving up to $300 a month—Excuse me! That's the car payment plus the electric bill—in order just to finance an infant's college education in 18 years.

At the same time, opportunities for entrepreneurial geniuses and hard-working stiffs alike are declining rapidly, as cash gets lost in a deficit crunch that's only beginning to flex its soul-destroying muscle. Optimism in the face of these realities is a lunatic's luxury.

The bottom line? Men who are now 30 to 50 years old are the first U.S. generation ever to be less successful than their fathers were at the same age—or, to put it another way, the first generation to fail at life.

TRUE ANXIETY THREE:
WOMEN HATE YOU

A good, stressless working environment is hard to find. We've talked about the shrinking job market and the shrinking paycheck. Now it's time to look at the shrinking tolerance of men by women. In some companies, the state of relations between the sexes is just short of hysterical. In the last two years the number of sexual harassment complaints has nearly doubled (including, as fans of Michael Crichton know, a boost in complaints by occasionally preyed-upon male employees).

Now, some psychologists theorize that in the deep, dark recesses of our subconscious, we blame females—along with a welter of policies aimed at addressing perceived social injustices—for swiping our jobs.

Can a woman cost you your job? That depends on your field and on the policies of the company you work for. Trouble is, you can't kid around about it, and you certainly can't make a date to talk about it later over dinner and drinks. There is serious, often unpleasant, confusion in what is right and wrong in dealing with female colleagues. "Even men who are hip and want to do the right thing aren't sure what you can and can't say, what constitutes sexual harassment," says Kenneth Wetcher, M.D., a Houston-based psychiatrist who specializes in men's issues. "The men I see are clearly confused and to some degree scared."

TRUE ANXIETY FOUR: LOVE STINKS

Amazing how many men's stressors have something to do with women. Actually, what's even more amazing is that we keep coming back for more. Not content with losing to women in the job market and in sexual-harassment court, we just can't help hoping that the best way to insure ourselves against the ugly stresses of life with women is to marry one. Weird, eh? Well, actually, a marriage that works is a proven stress-reliever. But for many of us, bringing a woman into our home is like calling Domino's and having them deliver an extra-cheese stress pie with bonus anchovies.

Take the two-career marriage. Most of us need one of these just to shore up our bank accounts against the rising tide of debt. But when both partners are working, who plays domestic? Who does all that stuff from diaper changing to laundry to washing dishes? You share it, right? Well, that's not how women see it, Buster. The people who monitor these things say that while we men have upped our "household help quotient," we still do only about half as much homework as our mates. So there's stress involved, since men feel like we've changed. Women, on the other hand, feel as if nothing has changed. Both are right. But she's madder.

Or take the one-career marriage, for that matter. Dr. Berglas tells the story of a couple who recently visited him for counseling. Both successful executives, they met, married and unexpectedly conceived a child in a matter of months. Then she quit her job to stay home and do the traditional thing, while he went on to conquer the world. When he landed a mammoth job promotion, she became resentful. "I never bought into being the senator's wife," she told Dr. Berglas bitterly. The result of such perceived imbalances? Maybe a temporary break-up. Maybe a permanent one. Fifty percent of marriages end in divorce. And nothing can match a divorce in progress for stress.

TRUE ANXIETY FIVE: YOU'RE OVERWIRED

Want to visit stress in its natural habitat? Take an unescorted walk through the Internet—and pay the connect charges yourself. Call it technostress, but our robots are in revolt. What has the on-line age done for us? We're on call (and worse yet, reachable) 24 hours a day. Every hour at work is matched by another hour lost to e-mail memos and fax retrieval. "We are being bombarded on a daily basis with much more than we can handle," warns Dr. Wetcher. "We have the technical ability to accomplish a lot more, but not the physical ability."

As for getting out of the fast lane, no exit. For men especially, the communication gizmos, which started as cool power status symbols of the '80s, have ended up as indispensable tools of the '90s. Plumbers have fax machines and car phones.

The avalanche of gadgetry, of course, is only symptomatic of the mayhem that passes for modern life. Look around you. Count the flashing LEDs. Those are the thousand points of light most of us see every day in a world filled to overflowing with new and improved stuff.

TRUE ANXIETY SIX: YOU'RE OVERWORKED

Psychologists say we are losing leisure time, not gaining it, as the conventional wisdom once held. More Americans are moonlighting than ever before. The average two-week work vacation in the United States pales in comparison to the six- and eight-week breaks common in northern Europe. Because our coping mechanisms for stress are, on average, much less effective than females', we need regular, active outlets. Traditionally, that wasn't a problem. Guys went bowling and played poker out of biological necessity, and their wives left them alone. Now there isn't time for such pleasant affectations. We're bone-tired and many of us are near burnout. "In 20 years of psychiatry, I can't recall a time when more men said they were tired and didn't have enough time," says Mark Unterberg, M.D., a Dallas-based psychiatrist. "Increasingly younger and younger men, guys in their thirties and forties, talk wistfully about retirement."

TRUE ANXIETY SEVEN: YOUR KID ISN'T CUTE

My friend Steve has never exactly been Mr. Relaxed, but now he's the father of a colicky newborn named Kathryn. When he returns home from 12-hour workdays, the baby wails. All night. He wants to be involved, supportive, the kind of hands-on dad he thinks his father wasn't, but he's got to get some sleep. His job, you see, is a hectic nightmare—lots of pressure, lots of stress.

Recently, when his wife stopped by the office to show off their seven-week-old girl, Kathryn screamed, and his co-workers went ballistic. The next week the Baby Kathryn Rule was imposed: No babies in the office.

Problem: While the fathering ideal has changed (and is in itself new, complicated and often mystifying, stress-inducing territory), corporate culture hasn't. An overwhelming number of men still believe that things like formal paternal-leave policies and flextime are frowned upon by their superiors and come at the expense of future job advancement. Many men believe that if they put their families first, they may jeopardize their jobs. Michael Kimmel, a sociologist at State University of New York at Stony Brook who writes about men's efforts to redefine themselves in his forthcoming book, *Manhood*, says that in corporate America the perceived cost of being a good father includes loss of income, male comradeship and manhood. "The definition of masculinity has proved remarkably inelastic," he writes. "Except for a few involved fathers, it binds men as tightly as ever to success in the public sphere, in the world of other men, as the markers of manhood and success."

TRUE ANXIETY EIGHT: WE'RE ALL GOING TO DIE

Woody Allen probably said it best: "It's not that I'm afraid to die. I just don't want to be there when it happens." Of course, aging is no joke. What we know is what happens as we *approach* the end point. Namely, our lung capacity deflates, muscle mass declines, bones weaken and joints begin to get arthritic. But what really bothers us most is regret at letting our prime-time years lapse, never having done anything meaningful, headline-making or what one friend calls the stuff to tell your grandchildren about.

Notes Robert Sapolsky, author of a smart, well-researched guide to stress and stress management called *Why Zebras Don't Get Ulcers*: "Mostly it's that aching sense that just when we finally grow up and learn to like ourselves and to love and play, the shadows lengthen." As we male Baby Boomers approach 50, it's easy to feel that our day of reckoning is at hand.

TRUE ANXIETY NINE: BUT WE WON'T BE THE FIRST TO GO

Of course, if we'd stop thinking about ourselves for a minute, we might be able to spot an even more serious cause of the kind of stress associated with aging: Not only are we going to die, but our parents are going to die first. Here's the

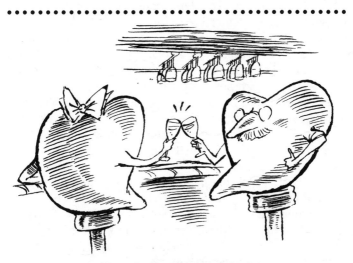

The Great White Hope

It's fairly well-known that drinking red wine in small quantities may help ward off coronary artery disease. But a study of nearly 82,000 men and women at Kaiser Permanente Medical Center in Oakland, California, concluded that white wine seems to do the job at least as well as red. Don't misunderstand. We're talking sipping here, not guzzling. Study leader and cardiologist Arthur L. Klatsky, M.D., stressed that these findings are in no way meant to encourage nondrinkers to start drinking, but he added, "for those who already drink, there is no health reason to stop, as long as you keep it to no more than two drinks per day. It might even do some good."

news: Our parents are older than we are. For an entire lifetime, that very fact was both their charm and their downside. Their persistent presence served to make many of us get out and get on our own as soon as possible.

But no matter how self-sufficient many of us are, the incipient death of a parent comes like a trumpet in the night to tell

. . . .

WORK IT OFF: BEST ANTI-STRESS MOVES TO HELP DEFUSE TENSION FAST

What do you do when your boss tosses another project in your lap and says he needs it tomorrow or some jerk sideswipes your new car or you're arranging parcels by ZIP code and a customer walks into your place of work *demanding* a book of stamps! The things that get our blood boiling often arise out of the blue. What we need is a way to cool down quickly before we see red.

The four stretches below will relax your body and calm your mind. But before you try them, you need to stand up and walk away from the problem for a few seconds. That's right, get away and get some air. "Anxiety produces a smothering feeling," explains Robert S. Brown, M.D., Ph.D., clinical professor of psychiatric medicine at the University of Virginia in Charlottesville. And among the causes is a drop in your body's store of carbon dioxide. Since normal breathing requires a sufficient carbon dioxide level in order to provide our bodies with enough oxygen, the rapid, shallow breaths we take when we're stressed actually deliver less oxygen to the blood and to the brain than regular breathing.

To get back to normal, concentrate on taking slow, easy breaths. Allow your abdomen, not your chest, to expand outward as you slowly inhale through your nose. Hold your breath for three to five seconds, then exhale slowly and completely through your lips before taking another deep breath.

Another pointer: Stand up. Slouching when stressed restricts breathing and circulation and can magnify feelings of helplessness.

When you've gotten your breathing under control, try the following exercises recommended by former world-class track-and-

. . . .

us we're really on our own. Once Mom goes, there's nobody else on Earth who *has* to love you, no matter what. No Boomer rites of passage, no amount of mind-numbing self-helpery can reduce the sadness we feel when nursing homes, powers-of-attorney and hospital visits all become the grim landmarks of a parent's final years.

• •

field athlete Greg Herzog in his book *The 15-Minute Executive Stress Relief Program*.

Neck. This is often the first place stress will appear, so Herzog recommends a two-point attack.

1. Reach with your right hand over your head and behind your left ear, grasping your neck. Pull your head gently toward your right shoulder. Then use your left hand to pull your head toward your left shoulder.

2. Clasp your hands behind your head with your elbows flared. Tilt your head forward so your chin is nearly touching your chest. Relax in this position for 30 seconds. Then slowly push your head up while resisting the movement with your clasped hands. When you finish, your head should be tilted back so you're looking at the ceiling.

Chest/Shoulders/Arms. Stand up straight with your arms extended in front of you, palms up. Bend your left arm at your elbow so your hand is pointing straight up. Then cross your right arm over to your left, grasping it just above the elbow. Now, push your left elbow away from your body while at the same time resisting the motion with your right arm. Hold the position for five to ten seconds, then repeat, using the other arm.

Back/Hamstrings. Stand with your feet shoulder-width apart and slowly bend forward, keeping your knees slightly bent so your lower back isn't strained. Let your upper body hang down with your arms extended toward the floor. Don't bounce or lock your knees. Relax your neck, letting your head hang down. Hold for 15 to 20 seconds, then slowly return to an upright position.

• •

TRUE ANXIETY TEN: YOU MAY NEVER HAVE SEX AGAIN

You want to go to the stress hall of fame? You want to take all your petty, Little League stresses about jobs and money and mortality and go right to the source of all adult male anxiety? Imagine penis death. Imagine the old guy just lies down and never gets up again. And imagine every woman you ever knew is watching it happen.

Every man alive has experienced a sudden and unexplained wilting, such as when he realizes just how big those latex condoms really are. For most of us, it's just a passing disaster, a temporary trauma, a little preview of personal apocalypse. At a certain age, however, it's the kind of fear that begins to grow. And if we're not fixating on the big fear—permanent impotency—there's the slightly less acute fear that our sexual stamina is on the wane and that our ability to satisfy our partner is just plain weakening.

But wait—isn't sex supposed to be the greatest of all stress-relievers? Not any more, it isn't. Aside from all the self-imposed performance stuff, sex now suffers from external pressures. For one, there's the threat of terminal illness. For the first time since the discovery of penicillin, a man can screw himself to death in one, brief unprotected moment. For another, there's the intrinsic seriousness of sex itself in these peculiarly puritanical times. For single men especially, what was once the ultimate relaxant is now just another stressor, the kind of thing that, in the hands of the right lawyer, can cost you your job, your fortune, your reputation and your freedom.

So, are stressors everywhere? Are we all simply a big, metaphorical snowball on the slippery slope of life, weighted with burdens and picking up more, whizzing downhill out of control? Not exactly. Gender anxiety, role changes, societal shifts may be unsettling, say stress experts, but they needn't be fatal. We men are becoming more willing to admit we don't have all the answers and rely on others for help, and to manage stress by better defining what we can and can't control, what we can and can't predict.

We are, in short, adapting. "Traffic jams, money worries, overwork, the anxieties of relationships . . . in our privileged lives we are uniquely smart enough to have invented these stressors and uniquely foolish enough to have let them, too often, dominate our lives," writes Sapolsky. "Surely we have the potential wisdom to banish their stressful hold."

—Todd Balf

Lighten Up Your Life

Did you ever wonder if you could get through the day without stepping on one of life's land mines? Here are 32 ways to deal with life's hassles.

• • • • • • • • • • • • • • • • • • •

AMERICA IS THE LAND OF melancholy invention. For a country so concerned about hygiene and landfills, we certainly seem to spend more than our share of time down in the dumps. For instance, Americans bereft of opportunity invented the blues, while Americans bereft of intelligent speech invented the bummer.

Sure, we have nearly unlimited access to clergymen and psychologists. And, yeah, yeah, we're all living longer and we're all boating more than ever and TV just gets "better" all the time. But we can't help it. Tension and bummage are everywhere.

In some ways it's not our fault. We're driven mad by the need to compete, by the unreasonable complexities of modern life, by unceasing demands on our time, by a planetful of dread and disease, by a boss with bad breath. We're victims. We're stressed. We're depressed.

Well, it's time to lighten up. Sure, that means setting aside your pre-occupation with the fascinating life and incredible times of Mr. Numero Uno, but the benefits of stress-busting, of lightening up under pressure, are so far-reaching they even outstrip the charms of self-absorption.

Research shows that while having a positive attitude and a sense of humor won't necessarily cure disease, it can keep you from getting sick and make you feel better, both emotionally and physically.

You don't believe it? Well, just consider the physiological effects of a good laugh. After a slight rise in heart rate and blood pressure, there's an immediate recoil.

Muscles relax, blood pressure drops below pre-laugh levels, and the brain releases endorphins, the same stress-reducing chemicals that are triggered by exercise. All this can help your body cope with difficult situations that typically stress the heart, not to mention the soul.

Unless you're one of those inanely grinning, psychotic optimists, lightening up is a learned skill. We spoke to professionals in a number of fields—from humorists skilled in breaking us up to psychologists who specialize in keeping us together—and asked them how they handle conflict while holding on to their sense of humor.

Here are some of their suggestions.

MARITAL MISERY

Conflict is inevitable in a marriage, especially in a new one. But counselors and psychologists have long known that knock-down-drag-out yelling matches can eventually kill a relationship. The key is to smooth out the ripples before they become tidal waves, says Craig W. Smith, Ph.D., director of the marriage and family therapy program at the University of Nebraska-Lincoln. Here's how.

Don't roll and run. Guys tend to roll their eyes, say "Here we go again" and retreat to the workshop in the basement when their wives get angry. Instead, sit down and hear her out.

Admit that you're wrong—even if you're not. "One of the best things you can do is simply say, 'Oops, I goofed,'" says Dr. Smith. "Directing humor at yourself, we've found, is an important way to defuse marital conflicts." Once you both calm down, you can reassess where the blame lies—and maybe get some justice.

Take the fight to another ring. Long, loud arguments often become circular—they go nowhere. If this happens, change locations; go to a coffee shop or restaurant or out on the front porch. "Sometimes taking the argument someplace new puts it in a different context and immediately deflates it," says Dr. Smith.

Walk away from the heat. Sometimes storming out is the right thing to do—with one caveat. Before you go, designate a time to talk it over after you've both calmed down. Say "I'll be back at two o'clock; we'll finish this then." Now you're free to go out and head-butt some masonry or chop some wood for a while.

Step gingerly on Wednesday. Couples fight most on Wednesdays and least on Thursdays, according to research at the University of Iowa in Iowa City. The reason: Wednesday is furthest from the weekend in both directions, making it the toughest day to get through. So Wednesday seems like an especially good day to leave job troubles at your office and bring home flowers instead.

Schedule weekly battles. By setting up a regular time every week (how about Thursdays?) to voice concerns and complaints, it's likely that you'll avoid bickering altogether. The idea is to head off skirmishes by talking about issues in a controlled, structured way.

NAKED STRESS

You've spent the whole day earning, achieving, creating and repairing—in short, doing all those things expected of a man. And doing them quite well, we might add. So why does sex—the fun part—so easily become a tension zone?

"For so many men, the big problem is that they make sex an extension of their eleven o'clock business meeting," says Michael Seiler, Ph.D., coauthor of the book *Inhibited Sexual Desire*. "It's a performance thing; it's work instead of pleasure. That kind of setting breeds anxiety."

Putting a little effort into lightening up under the covers, according to Dr. Seiler, can boost arousal and make sex even better.

Focus on having fun. By being aware that this is an experience about pleasure, not performance, you can begin to relax, says Dr. Seiler: "Concern yourself only with what feels good right now; then you'll get away from the question, 'What should I do?'"

What to do when you don't want sex but she does? "Just because you're not hungry, that doesn't mean you can't make her a sandwich," Dr. Seiler says. "Maybe you wouldn't mind kissing, touching or masturbating her. The idea is to be much more free and open to talk about things like this."

What to do when you want it and she doesn't? Oops, now we're getting personal. But if you're still reading, let's start with what *not* to do. And that is make her feel bad. Don't withdraw; ask her what she'd like to do. Or suggest a little intimacy without intercourse. Tell her, "Okay, let's just cuddle on the couch." That may be enough to change her mind, but if it doesn't, don't sweat it. There'll be other times.

Plan a little. "Sex can't always be a wild, spontaneous event," says Dr. Seiler. "If you wait for that to happen, you might be waiting a long time." So sometimes you have to schedule time for sex, even if it means getting up an hour early or hiring a babysitter.

MORNING MAYHEM

Sometimes stress just reaches out and grabs us when we're off guard. Like when we're stumbling out of bed with a straight razor in one hand, looking for a misplaced pair of glasses. If you don't blossom well in the first light of life's chaos, a stress-filled morning can ruin you for the rest of the day. Besides laying out your clothes the night before, what can you do to make the run smoother?

Follow the demands of your personality. "People who wake up and are fully charged and ready to go often make a mistake by sitting down to read the paper or watch the news," says Pamela Kristan, a time-management consultant for The Practical Matters in Boston. That's like downshifting. She suggests instead that you do something creative, whether it's playing with the kids or working out a strategy for a business meeting. That way you'll keep your energy high and leave the house feeling like you've already done something constructive. On the other hand, if you sort of ooze off the mattress and into the shower, you're probably better off sticking to a dull morning routine.

Get the sequence right. In fact, for many men—fast starters and early dawdlers alike—routine is everything, the desk organizer of a messy morning. There's a reason for this: By the time you kick, say at age 75, you've had breakfast 27,375 times. Pretty soon, maybe sometime around the 6,500th bowl of Wheaties, you figure out how to have breakfast the way you like it. If you make enough rituals, eventually, you'll find a place for everything, from coffee to crosswords. Invariably, a harried morning rush is the result of some significant change in your circumstances. Maybe you picked up a wife along the way. One day you get up and see that all your rituals have gone the way of your socks and underwear. What to do? Make new rituals, fast; experiment. Make a two-week commitment to do stretching exercises every morning. If it seems like the other events of the morning start to fall into place around that routine, stick to it. If you've always been a jump-out-of-bed-and-into-the-shower kind of guy, but that doesn't seem to work any more, reverse everything: Get up, eat, read the paper, exercise, *then* lather up. If after two weeks you're not satisfied with any new routine, try something different. The important thing to remember is, once something starts to work, don't change a thing. Become a slave to your new ritual. Be obsessed. This is the kind of eccentricity that makes wives crazy, by the way, but you can make up for it by delivering plenty of good, nutritious, stress-free sex.

OCCUPATIONAL THERAPY

From a psychological point of view, work is nothing but organized stress, so unless you work as a coma monitor in a small-town hospital, on the job is where you feel life pressing down most heavily and where you most feel a need to lighten up. Once you get to work, try these tactics to help lighten up your day.

Get your priorities right. Many people are overwhelmed by their jobs. They go into an office or factory and see one big wall of work ready to come crashing down on them. In fact, no matter how much pressure your job involves, you're only going to be able to do so much in an eight- or ten-hour day. By making sure you do the most important stuff first, you can lift some of the weight off your shoulders. "Be ruthless about cutting things out," says Kristan. Quickly list the tasks ahead of you, then compare them to each other. Is A more critical than B? Compare the winner to C, and so on until only the most essential task is left. Then get cracking.

Take the eagle's view. In the morning, at midday and an hour before you leave, step back and assess what you've accomplished and what needs to be done. Devise a trick to help change your point of view—walk to the other side of your office, or talk to yourself, or do a light stretching exercise. Anything to break whatever rut you might have gotten into.

Don't put off until tomorrow what can be completely ignored forever. Just realize that there are certain tasks you're never going to get to. Make a solid decision that you're going to figure out what they are and assiduously not do them. It's the only way to control the creeping scourge of inadequate time.

Get a new perspective on competition at work. "We've turned the workplace into a battle zone," says C. W. Metcalf, the author of *Lighten Up: Survival Skills for People under Pressure*, who runs humor-training programs for corporations. "Listen to them talk: 'The competition is *killing* us,' 'Our *mission* is . . . ,' 'I'd *die* for that promotion.' I mean, come on guys, where do you keep the howitzer?"

To lighten up at work and be able to defuse potential skirmishes with humor, Metcalf says, you need to "remain fluid and creative under pressure." To set the stage for cooperation, he counsels that you not tolerate isolation from your co-workers. According to Metcalf, feuds will keep simmering if all your contacts with office mates consist of memos and voicemail. A good manager will create programs that foster staff unity, but if yours doesn't, take the initiative. Organize a group lunch or some other activity, like a company softball team or Super Bowl pool. This approach has the added benefit of lightening up the boss, too. If he sees everyone else having fun, he's likely to want to join in.

There's life after work. Try to remember that others have a life outside the office, too. Jim Morris, a political humorist and impressionist who studies men in power, suggests that if you have a face-off with the boss, "remember that he's wearing his game face, the one we all bring to tough situations. If he has children, try to imagine him with his kids, or with his wife." If you can mentally strip away his hard-nosed image, you're more likely to stay calm yourself.

Help others find the humor in stressful situations. Don't be afraid of a witty remark. For example: If Joe down the hall says, "If I don't get this report done today, I'll shoot myself," ask him to leave a little note on his desk about the disposition of his stereo equipment—assuming you both don't work for the postal service. Most situations can be lightened with a self-deprecating joke, or one about the IRS.

Take a walk. And on the walk, think about everything in your life that makes you feel good: reading to your kids, a great beer, watching Dirty Harry movies.

Just because life's a game, don't be afraid to win. "The happiest people I know love to win," Metcalf says, "but it doesn't kill them when they lose."

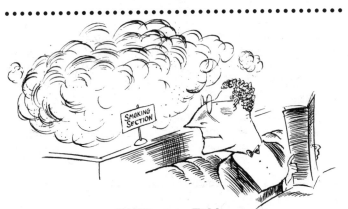

Waiting on Tables

Is it really worth waiting an extra ten minutes while the maître d' finds you a seat in the nonsmoking section of your favorite restaurant? In assessing air quality of seven restaurants, researchers found that the nicotine content in the air was 65 percent lower, on average, in the nonsmoking section than it was in the smoking section.

PUBLIC PRESSURE

If you want to see stress stand up and take a bow, put it at the podium in front of a bunch of strangers. Even if we aren't on the luncheon circuit, we all have our share of performance anxiety—whether it's while we're making a presentation of the company's annual report or asking a question at the local school board meeting. The sensation is the same: You open your mouth, and a small puff of dust settles on your audience.

"What most people forget is that when you give a presentation, your audience wants you to do well," says Neil Wilkinson, president of Toastmasters International, an organization dedicated to improved public speaking. "They're not there to try to pick you apart." Here are some of Wilkinson's insider tips on being calm in the eye of the storm.

Your degree of preparation runs parallel to your degree of relaxation. Know what you're going to say long before you open your mouth—and practice saying it out loud.

Humor can be your weapon, but don't force it. The best humor comes from personal anecdotes or funny tales related to the topic at hand—they make better ice breakers than that Eddie Murphy gag you've been saving. If life's been really boring lately, and you're really desperate for a laugh, you can crib stories from Comedy on Call, which supplies jokes, funny intros and closing remarks, and roast material for speakers by phone, fax or newsletter for a fee. For information, call 1-800-929-4269. For an immediate punch line, call 1-900-438-5284; it costs $1.50 a minute.

If you're caught off guard by a question, don't rush to fumble out some words. Take a deep breath, stand up, repeat the question—whatever it takes to buy yourself some time

• •

Kids: Resource or Drain?

A father's relationship with his children has a strong bearing upon his physical and mental health, according to one study. The more aggravation you get from your kids, the more likely you'll be popping Tums. On the other hand, the joys of harmonious fatherhood can help you cope with the stresses of life. The key, it seems, is getting your little tax deductions to recognize when their therapeutic presence is needed—and when the football game is on.

to formulate an answer. Also there's the ultimate, honorable fallback: "I don't know." It's amazing how well people respond to honesty.

Finally, heed some famous advice. Wilkinson recommends Winston Churchill's saying that if you're nervous about speaking to a roomful of people, simply imagine them all naked. But don't stare at that redhead in the third row.

PROBLEM CHILDREN

Maybe at work you can handle even the most stressful moments with the grace of a professional. Your kids don't care. Your most shining moment may be saving the company a $100 billion contract. To your kids, it's how well you play pile-of-dogs or how scary you can make a bedtime story. Making that kind of shift is difficult, especially for those guys who work under pressure all day.

"A lot of men have trouble making the transition from work to fathering," concedes Jerrold Lee Shapiro, Ph.D., professor of counseling psychology at Santa Clara University in California and author of *The Measure of a Man*. "At work, what's important is the doing. At home, it's the being." Here are some of his suggestions for being a friend as well as a father without losing your authority-figure status.

Don't play Mr. Fix-It. "Remember that children learn by trying things, not by being shown," says Dr. Shapiro. Even if you show them a better way, they're going to want to experiment. So don't get uptight if they don't follow your instructions.

Schedule some fun. You need to plan time with your kids just as you would a tennis game or an important meeting at work.

Don't split your time. Make a commitment not to try to do anything else when you're with your kids. "Spending time with the kids does not mean playing with them during time-outs in the football game," says Dr. Shapiro. That will only leave both of you frustrated.

Set rules for guests. Especially if your child has playmates visiting, remind him of the house rules before the friends come over. That way you've enlisted him to help supervise play, and with any luck you won't have to get involved, Dr. Shapiro says. "Of course, if the neighbor's kid comes over and starts playing with the chain saw, this approach may need to be modified."

Tread softly with teens. When it comes to teenagers, things get tricky, since teens live in a stress warp, where emotions and feelings are magnified by a factor of ten. "Don't start a conversation by asking them something like, 'How's it going at school?'" Dr. Shapiro says. That's death. He advises, instead, the unthinkable: talking a little about yourself. "I don't mean your inner feelings or anything like that, just something like what you did at work that day. It can help defuse the natural tension." The idea here is to humanize yourself, since teenagers often cease viewing their fathers as sentient beings.

FAMILY FOLLIES

Maybe you dread talking to your in-laws because they always bring up your wife's former boyfriend, the handsome attorney who's now running for the state house. Or maybe you dread talking to them because they don't speak English or because they fling small bubbles of saliva from between their teeth. The Bulgarian dialect and the shower-talk may be things you're powerless to help. But the gratuitous insults are a little more manageable. "You can prepare yourself for those zingers that make you steam," says psychologist Leonard Felder, Ph.D., author of *Does Someone at Work Treat You Badly?* "When one comes, say to yourself, 'Bingo, there it is, no visit would be complete without it.' That'll turn it into something funny in your mind and keep you from getting angry."

Not all of us are so great at reining in our tempers, of course, so take some precautions to keep yourself from getting riled. Here are a few suggestions on how you can keep the fat from hitting the fire.

Give the gift of humor. A funny book or videotape or tickets to a comedy show can take the edge off. "Make it something you can share together," says Joel Goodman, Ed.D., director of the HUMOR Project in Saratoga Springs, New York. "Laughter's a terrific bonding device."

Ask for help. It could be anything from fixing the sink to investing in stocks to the right way to brush the dog, just as long as it distracts them from offering advice on everything else you do.

Find out what you have in common. Maybe it's bass fishing with your father-in-law or watching James Cagney movies with your wife's mom. Probably the most universal unifying element is grandchildren. Plan your outings with your kids and their grandparents. "Plan" is the operative word here. If you remain in control, you have the best shot at remaining stress-free.

A final bit of advice: Look for the land mines, so you see them before you step on them. Some situations are unavoidably stressful. You can't take an airplane, perform brain surgery, file for divorce or bungee jump without a little flutter of stress, right? But much of what causes stress in our lives comes from things we could easily avoid without sacrificing our reputations or our responsibilities. There's no law that says you have to drive 70, that's for sure. And the secret grudge you've been nurturing since college isn't a great souvenir. Sometimes, it seems our lives are so stressful, we don't notice how much stress-junk is there by invitation. The solution is to clean up. Then lighten up.

—Jeff Stevenson

Sailing Away

Boating combines a lot of hard work, brushes with danger, awe-inspiring beauty and expensive equipment. So what are you waiting for?

• • • • • • • • • • • • • • • • • •

IN THE END, it's a testosterone thing, like big muscles and hunting, and—if we're to face facts—the losing of the hair. Somewhere down in the genetic memory of the sex, men have been programmed with a basic desire to boat.

We get a rush out of putting our hands on the levers of a

powerboat's throttle and imagining something 500 times the size of a self-propelled lawn mower begin to move beneath us. We like to wander through the boat shows and point out to the little woman how everything has to be stored just so, because if it isn't, and the weather kicks up, well, you get the idea.

Indeed, boating remains one of the last fundamentally male pursuits that women haven't yet invaded—and they're not likely to anytime soon, either. If you look through the boating magazines these days, you'll undoubtedly encounter increasing references to "quality time" in the marketing campaigns of America's $9-billion-a-year pleasure-boat industry. The ads usually picture fathers and their smiling families all grinning at each other as that 28-foot "Mediterranean cruiser" carves a vee through water so blue that it probably can't even be found in Al Gore's dreams.

But don't be fooled. What's really going on in these ads is that the boatbuilder is inviting you to join him in a plot against the little woman. The idea? To convince her that it's okay for you to buy the boat—in fact, that you must buy the boat, because without the boat there just may not be any quality time! In short, that you really will take the wife and kids along with you every summer weekend for the next 20 years, and that there really will be enough room aboard a vessel resembling an oversize Clorox bottle with the interior dimensions of a walk-in closet for two adults and two children to get away from it all and still be smiling—just like in the ads—once there's no land in sight anywhere.

WOMEN HATE BOATS

The ads don't tell the truth, and the truth is this: Women hate boats. Okay, not all women, but how about most? Ask around and see for yourself. They hate the way boats smell—especially after the Port-a-pottie starts misbehaving. They hate the way the food spoils too fast and the way everything feels cramped. But above and beyond everything else, they hate the ever-present sense of impending doom, as in the boat's going to sink or blow up or the kids will fall off or you will fall off—and then she'll have to take the wheel and actually start looking for you (because when you're 60 miles out in the Gulf Stream, you can't just "pull over" and wait for help).

And yet what men like most of all is the very thing about

boating that terrifies women—the idea that casting off from the dock amounts to nothing less than the willful and gratuitous placing of one's self in harm's way, like driving a race car or fighting a bull or moving to Los Angeles.

In the same way that guys in Porsches always flash their headlights when passing in the street, or that men with mustaches invariably make eye contact with each other when passing on the sidewalk, guys who are into boats share a secret that even they don't fully understand: That in their own quiet way, they too have courted death and lived to tell about it—just like Danny Sullivan or Sir Edmund Hillary.

One might object that taking a 25-foot day sailer into Long Island Sound on a summer Sunday is not quite the same as climbing Mount Everest. But when that little puff of mid-morning cloud grows into a late-day thunderhead that starts hurling golf ball–size hailstones and forked lightning at you along with 60-mile-an-hour winds that come up out of nowhere, well, when something like that happens, you might well prefer to be 20,000 feet above sea level saying good-bye to your Sherpa guides.

So, given all the forgoing, the question is this: If you're not one of nearly 14 million American males who already own one, is there a boat in your future? And if so, what should it be?

The sailboat market collapsed in the 1980s as suddenly-rich young professionals began gravitating to the less nautically arcane world of powerboating. Since then, the price of sailboats has gone from bad to worse (or good to better, depending on which side of the cash register you're on). Result: You can currently buy a new 35-foot sloop with all the amenities of a vacation cabin in the woods—shower, stove, fridge, toilet and hot and cold running water—for well under $80,000. For a similarly equipped vessel in good condition on the used-boat market, prices can dip well below $50,000.

You can find equally big bargains in the powerboat market. Boats that cost $150,000 new five years ago can today be bought in "Bristol condition" (that's boat-world jargon for tip-top shape) on the used-boat market for half that price. Lower-priced boats have experienced equivalent declines. Meanwhile, the price of gasoline and diesel fuel has leveled off, and marinas in many states are offering seasonal slips at deeply discounted prices as well.

But is owning a boat something you genuinely want to do? To help you decide, what follows is a six-point checklist of tips and warnings to take into account. Boating can be one of the great joys of male adulthood, but rush into it impulsively and you can torpedo the family budget, not to mention run the very real risk of getting yourself killed.

HOW BIG AND WHAT KIND?

The first thing to know is that the world of boats is divided in two—power and sail (aka "stinkpots" and "rag baggers")—and they are, well, like ships that pass in the night. Power-boaters—which as a group outnumber sailboaters at least two to one—dump on rag baggers for indulging in a method of transportation that can take all day to go half a mile if there's no wind. By contrast, sailboaters respond that powerboaters have noisy, polluting vessels that aren't boats any more so much as floating condos with interiors that sometimes look like Bangkok brothels, with mirrors and Formica in place of mahogany and other woods.

Forget all that and decide this way: How far do you want to travel on a weekend, and where will you keep the boat in the meantime? A sailboat that travels 6 knots (about eight miles per hour) is only going to cover a fourth of the distance, in the same period of time, as a powerboat that can plow ahead at 25

• •

Towel Trick

Everyone knows that white and other light colors reflect the sun's rays and dark colors absorb them. So why do they make ice chests and coolers dark green, blue and red? Beats us. But you can keep beer and food inside them colder longer—even through eight hours of direct Labor Day sun at the beach—with an old camping trick that requires only a beach towel and a white tablecloth. The first step is to soak the towel in water and drape it over the cooler. Next, put the tablecloth on top, tucking the ends under the corners so the wind won't blow it off. The white tablecloth will act as a reflector against the sun's rays, and the slow evaporation of the water in the towel will lower the temperature on the cooler's surface.

knots. Also, any relatively low-lying bridge will be an obstacle to a sailboat but most likely not to a powerboat.

HOW DO I LEARN TO BE AN OLD SALT?

Whether you decide on a sailboat or powerboat, it is essential to take a course in seamanship and small-boat handling. A good course will cover the basics of navigation, safety at sea, docking and anchoring, chart reading, the proper use of lines, the fundamentals of weather forecasting and so on.

CAN I REALLY AFFORD THIS?

Just as the major expenditures in the computer business can involve programming and software, the big bucks in boating are often spent on what you buy afterward to make the boat safe and usable. For example:

- No boat worthy of the name should be without a depth sounder, but a decent unit, say, the Humminbird HDR-200, can cost up to $270.

- A two-way VHF radio is also a must, and it won't come cheap, either. A good unit such as the Standard Horizon Eclipse can cost as much as $370.

- If you plan to go boating in any area that is prone to summer fogs, you should also consider investing in at least a small-boat "closed array" radar unit with a range of 16 miles. The best one available at the moment is the Raster Scan by Apelco, which can sell for over $2,000.

- If you plan to travel beyond the sight of land, a loran position-finder is a wise investment. These devices use radio signals received from government-maintained loran towers along the East, West and U.S. Gulf coasts to locate a boat's position on a nautical chart. A reliable loran by Raytheon can set you back about $1,000. Or for the ultimate in accuracy, you can spend $1,100 or more for a GPS (Global Positioning System) unit of the sort that the U.S. Army relied on to find its way around in Desert Storm.

Then, of course, you'll need charts to know where you are after the loran or GPS gives you the longitude and latitude coordinates, plus a pair of binoculars to see where you're going, as well as lines to anchor and dock with—to say nothing of countless other, less vital accessories to make the boat comfortable if you plan to stay on the water for more than a couple of hours each weekend. Add it all together and that three-year-old 25-foot Bayliner you've been eyeing at a price tag of $15,000 can easily turn out to cost $20,000 by the time you're ready to turn on the engine and cast off.

AM I HANDY WITH A SCREWDRIVER?

The marine environment is just about the harshest on Earth for almost anything man-made. As a result, everything on a boat ultimately breaks. If you wait for it to break before replacing or repairing it, you are asking for very big trouble, for the failure will almost assuredly come exactly when you need dependability the most.

Let's say you've applied that old landlubber's cliche—if it ain't broke, don't fix it—and failed to change the fuel filters on time. Then you get into rough seas that churn up the sediment at the bottom of the fuel tanks. Then the sediment moves through the fuel lines and clogs up the filters, starving the engines for fuel. And finally, there you are, lost at sea, with waves breaking all around and everyone feeling sick, and dammit, the boat just won't go and you don't know why. A little inconvenient, no?

In sum, if you're a mechanically minded kind of guy—someone who can actually get a stalled car to start instead of making the problem worse—then the maintenance tasks on a boat will be both challenging and fun. Anyone with a decent tool kit and a repair manual can maintain a boat engine. By contrast, if you're the kind of guy who likes to procrastinate, then forget about boating; psychologically, the maintenance chores will be a burden, and ultimately, you'll find a way to avoid doing them—at which point fate will take over.

AM I GRACEFUL UNDER PRESSURE?

When you're on the water, a crisis can arise at any time—and when it does, things can happen fast. So are you unflappably even-tempered yet forceful under stress? Or do you raise your voice and tell everyone to "Shut up, I've got to think!" when the three-year-old spills his milk? If the latter, then before you get into boating, seek professional help on why you're so wound up; in your present state, boating won't relax you, it'll bring out the worst of what's boiling up inside.

CAN I STAND NOT HAVING THE BIGGEST BOAT IN THE MARINA?

"Five-foot-a-year disease" is one of the most common maladies of pleasure boaters. It is caused by pursuing two equally unattainable goals: (a) to buy a boat big enough to reduce the sea to something as flat as the parking lot of a mall and (b) to own a boat so in-your-face huge as to be absolutely, positively guaranteed to be the biggest vessel in any marina you may ever visit.

In the lobby of the Forbes Building in New York City is a scale-model display of several boats, each progressively larger than the next. They illustrate what five-foot-a-year disease did to the late Malcolm Forbes. He began with a 72-foot Canadian Corvette power cruiser called Highlander, and finally wound up with a 151-foot steel-hulled vessel—Highlander V—that was built for him by a shipyard in the Netherlands.

Too bad for Malcolm, but scarcely had he taken delivery—laying brief but glorious claim to the title of being the owner of the biggest private yacht in New York harbor—when an even bigger New York show-off happened along. That person was Donald Trump, who bought and refurbished a yacht—Trump Princess—that was nearly twice the size of Highlander V. Then, of course, Trump went broke, the yacht was sold, and Malcolm's son, Steve, remains stuck with Highlander V. The moral? As any high-school boy will tell you, when it comes to size, there are other things to measure besides boats.

—*Chris Byron*

A Beginner's Guide to Golf

It's been called the world's most frustrating game.
Don't believe it for a minute. Here's our golf primer.

• • • • • • • • • • • • • • • • • • •

EVERY KID DREAMS OF being a sports hero. Who didn't once imagine he was Mickey Mantle, standing at home plate, or Jimmy Brown, charging through the line? But most of those dreams stay just that: dreams. Only a tiny fraction of us ever grow up to see one of our hits sail over the wall at Yankee Stadium or hear the roar of the crowd as we race across the mud in Cleveland. But when it comes to golf, you actually can go where your heroes go and (maybe) do what your heroes do.

On the Old Course at St. Andrews, Scotland, you place your tee in the same bit of ground as James Braid and Harry Vardon and old Tom Morris once did. At Pebble Beach in California, men like Nicklaus and Hogan and Palmer have faced the same first shot you do.

Okay, it's true that those great golfers ended up with better final scores than the average player could possibly hope for. But the other great thing about golf is that once or twice a round ... a month ... a year, every golfer somehow manages to hit a shot that turns out absolutely perfect. And every golfer, when he hits that drive right on the screws or that putt that moves inerrantly across the green and into the hole, knows in his heart that even the great Jack Nicklaus couldn't have done it better. Sure, golf has always had an air of snobbery about it, and for many men their performance on the golf course is mainly about toadying up to the board chairman. But for the true linksman, golf is more than a sport. Golf is in his blood. It's endlessly fascinating, mentally challenging, virtually unconquerable. If you haven't tried golf yet, here's what you need to know to get started.

THE EQUIPMENT

It's easy for a beginning golfer to get intimidated here. Take a look at any magazine and you'll be overwhelmed with ads from the dozens of club manufacturers touting their high-technology gear in the kind of complex jargon best reserved for a Ross Perot infomercial. But the fact is, buying a set of golf clubs does not require advanced degrees in metallurgy, aerodynamics or physics. Here are the few terms being used in golf equipment today that you really need to know, translated into normalspeak.

Cambered sole. The sole, or bottom, of the club is curved, which prevents it from digging into the ground and helps you avoid flop shots and stubs.

Cavity back. A design element for irons—also known as perimeter weighting—in which a cavity is formed on the back of the clubhead behind the center, allowing weight to be flared outward. This helps the clubhead remain more stable as it strikes the ball and directs more energy into shots hit off-center.

Flow weighting. In a set of irons, extra weight is shifted toward the toe (the outer end) of the clubface as the lofts of the club decrease. For example, there is more toe weight in a three-iron than in the nine-iron. This compensates for the tendency to contact the ball toward the toe when using longer irons.

Investment casting. This is a relatively new process used to make clubheads in which molten steel or metal alloy is poured into wax molds. Molds allow the designer the latitude to create specialized shapes—the cavity back is a perfect example—that once would have been impossible. The old style of club making, still in use, is forging, in which clubheads are stamped from solid chunks of steel.

Loft. This is the degree to which a clubface slants upward when squarely placed on the ground, the angle of which is measured in degrees. The degree of loft helps determine the steepness of a shot's trajectory, the distance it travels and how much backspin is imparted to the ball.

• •

Killer Golf

In Japan, golf is a killer. It has been reported that nearly 5,000 Japanese die every year on golf courses. Apparently, that's because the links are an extremely stressful place. Greens fees are expensive, you have to book your tee time months in advance and courses are so jam-packed with players that foursomes can be spaced as little as six minutes apart.

Progressive offset. A feature in some irons in which the shaft is set slightly ahead of the bottom line (or leading edge) of the clubface. It results from the curving of the neck (or hosel) of the clubhead and encourages golfers to keep their hands ahead of the clubface during the swing, a desirable practice. Because offset benefits longer more than shorter irons, club designers add progressively more from the wedge up to the three-iron.

Sweet spot. This is the specific point at the center of the clubface that applies the maximum distance, the optimum trajectory and a solid feeling when it hits the ball. With the perimeter-weighting designs, the sweet spot is effectively enlarged, just as in large-head tennis rackets.

GOOD CLUBS

It's one thing to know your golf jargon; it's quite another to get good clubs that'll serve you well. Tempted by those $179 special sets at K Mart? Hold yourself back. You should no more buy clubs off the rack without a proper fitting than you would purchase a suit without tailoring. Not only is every golfer a different height and weight, but each one swings the club in an individual way.

Many golf retail stores offer some kind of custom-fitting service. Some may charge $50 or so, but it's money well-spent. You can usually get the same service free at your local course's pro shop if you buy your clubs there. Here's a preview of what they'll be looking at.

Swing speed. How fast you swing the club determines what kind of shafts you should have. Generally, the faster you swing, the stiffer a shaft you need.

Lengths and lies. Some people swing more around, others up and down. And, obviously, everyone is a different height and has a different reach. These factors determine the proper length and lie (angle formed between shaft and bottom edge of the clubhead).

Grip size. The wrong grip can destroy your game. Oversize grips prevent proper hand rotation, leading to the dreaded slice. Undersize grips cause hands to rotate too quickly, leading to hooks.

The golf shaft may be the most important, yet most overlooked part of a beginning golfer's club purchase decision. The shaft is nothing but a thin tube, made of either stainless steel, titanium, aluminum alloy or graphite composites. In the transition between the slow backswing and the powerful forward swing, the shaft actually bends along its length and twists from side to side. A good shaft should snap back straight just at the moment of impact with the ball.

Shafts come in varying flexes, from stiff to regular to soft. In general, the stiffer the flex, the more clubhead speed is needed to make the shaft straighten out at impact—that's where you want it to be. Also, some are designed to flex lower down the shaft, near the clubface, while others bend higher up the shaft. A shaft with a low flex point usually results in a higher trajectory, a benefit for beginners or anyone with a weak swing since it helps get the ball higher in the air. Better players tend to prefer higher-flex-point shafts, which deliver more control.

Stainless steel shafts have been used in golf clubs predominantly since they replaced hickory shafts back in the 1920s. They're fine for beginners, but the new graphite shafts, some with carbon and boron filaments, are usually a few grams lighter in weight, allowing you to generate a faster swing. Also, graphite has the benefit of absorbing hand- and arm-jolting shocks and vibrations—especially welcome for golfers who practice frequently or mis-hit the ball.

THE SWING

Whole books have been written about the golf swing. The truth of the matter is that it's really not all that complicated. The key is getting balanced and set before you swing. As Jack Nicklaus says it: "If you don't have the proper grip and the proper set-up, I can't teach you how to swing or play the game." There are but four fundamentals that all good golf swings— and hence all good golfers—have in common.

Grip. Avoid a death grip that makes the tendons expand and the sweat begin to pour down the forehead. If you're holding the club as if you're trying to choke a snake, you're in trouble before you begin. Instead, the club should rest comfortably in the fleshy pads of the fingers, thumbs down the top of the shaft, fingers intertwining easily, palms facing each other. Take a lesson and have a Professional Golfer's Association (PGA) pro show you the correct position, or read Ben Hogan's book *Five Lessons*.

Alignment. Harvey Penick, a teaching pro now in his eighties, published a volume of tips called his *Little Red Book*. It's an excellent book about golf and life in general. And his number-one golf tip is take dead aim. It's simple, but most golfers don't pay heed. Getting properly aligned, which means making sure your feet, knees, hips and shoulders are all pointed in the same direction (perpendicular to the ball's line of flight), is critical to success in golf.

Stance. The spacing of the feet, the placement of the ball, your distance from the ball—get any one of these things out of whack and you'll be searching for your ball in the woods. Generally:

- Feet should be shoulder-width apart.

- The ball is usually played opposite the left heel (for righties), but can move back slightly for mid- to short-iron shots.

- When you set up for a practice shot with your arms in a natural position (i.e., relaxed, with elbows bent), the sole of the club should sit flat on the ground behind the ball.

Posture. Many golfers bend over too far or stand too erect. The posture most pros teach is a comfortable, athletic one with knees slightly flexed, feet comfortably apart, arms hanging down freely from the shoulders. Not sure if you have it right? Tip: Your weight should be on the balls of your feet.

The swing itself is a slow coiling motion in the backswing, followed by a forward release of energy through the ball, finishing off with a full follow-through. Simple enough, right? Back in the 1920s, one eccentric golf teacher told his students to just "swing the clubhead," which is to say, *don't* swing the shaft. The way to do that is to imagine the clubhead isn't attached to a rigid shaft at all, but instead to a handkerchief. His pupils were instructed to swing the clubhead backward and forward and just let the ball get in the way. This technique can help you get over the natural tendency to muscle the ball.

If you watch the professionals, you will notice one thing above all: tempo. The best players don't "hit" the ball. Rather, they swing with a relaxed, almost lazy rhythm, looking like they're just trying to make contact. Which, of course, is one of the secrets. Because when you make solid contact, even with a slow swing, the ball goes like a rocket. Some suggestions:

- The clubhead should make a circular path from beginning to end. If the club makes a figure eight in the air, the ball is heading for the woods.

- Don't worry too much about keeping your head down. This common bit of advice given to (and frequently by) beginners can, if taken too strictly, make you freeze up completely. That results in an arms-only swing, which won't do you much good. A little back-and-forth head movement is actually a good thing.

- Hit down to hit up. A frequent mistake is to swing with a scoopy, lifting stroke when you want the ball to go high. You should hit down and allow the angle of the clubface to send the ball high.

- Tape yourself. For the money, the best stroke-improvement device is impact tape, available in most golf shops. You stick the tape on the clubface and check the mark after your shot to see whether you heeled the ball, bladed it, topped it, toed it or hit it square in the center.

THE GAME

You'll need to take lessons, of course. But the key is practice. And our advice is: Spend your time wisely. Statistics show that in an average round of golf, only 53 percent of your score will consist of full-swing shots. That means 47 percent, or nearly half, of your score will be made up of putts; short shots around the greens such as chips, pitches and sand shots, and other recovery or half-swing shots.

The lesson is clear: If you want to lower your score, spend at least half your practice time on these more delicate shots, instead of just whacking at ball after ball.

(continued on page 101)

- -

WHAT IT COSTS TO BREAK 100
THE NEW GOLFER'S EXPENSE SHEET

You say your plan is to ascend the corporate ladder, and golf is the chosen vehicle. If you're sure you can devote the time it will take to advance from total nongolfer to high-90s shooter in a few months, that's terrific. You should set aside the money now.

Forgive us any insult to your sense of golf's nobility, but this accounting assumes that your actual goal is not golf mastery but image-enhancement and bonding with corner-office personnel. Therefore, we list only premium goods and services.

In sequence, then, neophytes, please obtain:

- A graphite-shafted driver with an oversize steel head. $230

- A 15-degree lofted fairway club, also graphite and steel. $180

- A very high lofted fairway club (seven-wood equivalent) with graphite shaft and rails on the sole. $180

- A set of steel-shafted, cavity-back irons of an *au courant* make and model like Tommy Armour 845s or Ping Zings; three-iron through PW (pitching wedge). $640

- Three head covers. Only the driver cover can be the stuffed-animal variety that's so in style. The other two can match each other, but all three shouldn't match. Don't ask why. $20

- A good sand wedge. Buy it separately from the other irons, from a driving range or golf superstore that will give you a free five-minute lesson in sand play with your purchase. $60

- A fancy putter—a Ping, perhaps, or one from the French-designed Taylor Made line. $70

- A nifty, "high-tech" nylon golf bag. Shop the knock-offs. $95

- Your first pair of spikes—water-resistant leather up-

- -

pers, white with black saddles; no kiltie, please, if you can resist it. $110

- Pullcart—don't buy one. Much hipper and more efficient to rent it for $3 a round. $20

- A good golf umbrella. (Sounds like a lot, but it's in lieu of an expensive rainsuit.) $40

- Three true golf shirts. Jacquard knit, banded sleeves, two buttons. $150

- Two pairs of golf slacks. Dockers are good. $85

- Golf socks. There are such things, but you should pretend there aren't. $0

- Cap. Wear your favorite logoed nongolf cap, avoiding auto parts and farm equipment companies. $0

- Sweaters. Wear what you have, in general, but succumb to one pro-shop beauty for "good luck." $75

- Golf glove (worn on left hand by righties). A white Foot-Joy Sta-Sof of Pittards cabretta leather will last you half a season. $19.00

- Bug spray, sunscreen, lip balm. Raid your medicine chest. $0

- Six lessons in series from an established local pro (taken with two soulmates who each pay one-third of the total $450 fee). $150

- Practice balls—enough to last over the course of 12 trips to the range. $90

- Stack of golf how-to magazines. $15

- *Golf My Way*, the Jack Nicklaus video. $60

- *Ben Hogan's Five Lessons* instruction book. $17

- Tees, Band-Aids, impulse items. $6

- 15-pack of no-cut golf balls. $21

• •

WHAT IT COSTS TO BREAK 100
THE NEW GOLFER'S EXPENSE SHEET—CONTINUED

- Green fee. Your first round ever at the local public course. $18

- Another 15-pack of balls. $21

- Green fee. Your second round (but highest score) ever at the local public course. $18

- Green fee, local course; score: 127. $18

- Green fee at the new upscale public course a half-hour away. $36

- Mandatory motorized cart fee. $12

- Green fee at the local course; you shoot 112. $18

- Green fee; you shoot 107. $18

- Green fee; score: 103. $18

- Balls. $21

- Green fee; you shoot a legitimate 97 with only a first-tee mulligan. Bravo. $18

Total cost: $2,549.00

Well, if you hadn't realized it before, taking up golf is a financially significant decision. You lay out money for those few items that you think will get you started; then it's funny (excuse me, sad) how quickly it adds up.

Still, if you treat the whole project as a calculated effort to move up in the world, the $2,000-plus investment—and the attendant challenge to your motor skills and grit—could easily prove profitable.

But please, if one day you start to see promise in yourself, if golf jargon begins to speckle your speech and golf collectibles catch your eye in resort-town storefronts, do not accuse the makers of this list of low-balling the cost of your new hobby. In cases where the purchase of a golf game is complete, the total cost spirals beyond your checkbook and stops on the far side of your soul.

• •

Next, learn the game's rules and etiquette.

Rules: Hit the ball with the club until you get it into the hole. That pretty much does it for rules.

Etiquette: Make sure you're ready when it's your turn, and make your shot quickly. Probably the biggest annoyance in golf is slow play. Watching Joe Weekender take three practice swings, then spend two minutes patting down microscopically out-of-place grass before making a three-foot putt is enough to make some players begin contemplating less sportsmanlike uses for their clubs. Some of this comes from the desire to emulate our weekend television heroes by taking lots of practice swings, lining up putts and other nonsense. If you want to emulate a golfing star, do like John Daly: Grip it and rip it!

Taking care of the golf course: replacing divots, raking bunkers and fixing ball marks in greens and so forth is also important. To get a free copy of the rules, including information on golf etiquette, write the U.S. Golf Association, Golf House, P.O. Box 708, Far Hills, NJ 07931.

One of the best tips ever given in golf was when a teacher explained that most people out for a round of golf aren't really playing golf... they're playing a game called "golf swing."

The secret of successful golf, if there is one, is not to think about weight shifts and supinated wrists but to concentrate on the target and how the ball should get there.

Sure, it sounds simple, but even the greatest golfers have days when they feel like wrapping their clubs around telephone poles. And maybe that's the magic of golf; no matter how good you get, the challenge will always continue.

A GOLF COURSE

There's nothing like a long weekend of totally focused attention to lift your game a notch or two. Following are five top golf schools.

Golf Digest Schools. Affiliated with the monthly magazine, these schools are held at selected resorts around the country. Call 1-800-243-6121.

John Jacobs Practical Golf Schools. Basic fundamentals-oriented program. Most sessions are held at Marriott golf resorts around the country. Call 1-800-472-5007.

Innisbrook Golf Institute. Part-time PGA Tour player Jay Overton directs this excellent school at a top-rated Florida resort. Call 1-800-456-2000.

The Ben Sutton Golf Schools. Another excellent basic program for all ages and levels of play. Sessions are in Florida. Call 1-800-225-6923.

Golf University at San Diego. Ken Blanchard adapts his *One-Minute Manager* theories to golf. At the Rancho Bernardo Inn. Call 1-800-426-0966.

—James Y. Bartlett

Part 4

MAN-TO-MAN TALK

How to Live Till
Your Next Birthday

*Are you taking teenage risks with a 40-year-old
body? Let one man's experience guide you toward
greater wisdom.*

• • • • • • • • • • • • • • • • • •

BAD OLD FATHER TIME, who uses a rigged deck, eventually nails everyone. If you're smart and play your cards right, you might stick around for a little while. But if you're careless, if you're stupid, if you hide in a young man's mind while your aging body grows breasts, Father Time and his sandbagging shill, Uncle Mortality, will take you to the cleaners. Take my word for it.

So it was that these two were with me on Christmas Eve Day, along with my nine-year-old son, as I faced the ski jump. Ahead was a steep 75-foot descent and a corresponding rise with a bulging lip at the top, the whole narrow trail resembling the spine of a swayback mare. As I looked down, that familiar tickle of vertigo electrified my scrotum, a survival of the species alarm that warned, "Danger, Will Robinson, Danger."

"Wow. It looks pretty hairy," my wise young son cautioned. Then he skied down to the bottom of the hollow and waited for me to do the same. But I heeded neither my boy nor the puny whimper of my testicles. Instead I was listening to Uncle Mo. *What? You've reached 40 and you're gonna stop living? You wanna skip something, make it dessert—but not this jump. I want to soar and you keep stepping on my cape!*

I pushed off, passed the blur of my son at the bottom, then screamed up the slick tongue of the path leading to the jump. Betting into my delusion, I crouched on my haunches for speed, then shot off the lip at the top. In the air I became weightless, the first indication that I had seriously violated the laws of nature. The next came when I hit the ground with such violence that it felt as if a giant hand was trying to force my entire body, head first, into an empty Vienna sausage can. Rolling and tumbling, I smacked the center of my back against a mogul. This instantly paralyzed me, and for the rest of my fall, my arms and legs bounced over the snowpack like delicatessen salamis.

I SAW MY FUTURE

As I lay motionless, I saw the future in the cool piety of white powder: the whooping ambulance that would take me down the mountain, the rotisserie-like contraption to which I would be pinioned when my grief-stricken, pale wife would see me. I saw the virile young man she would eventually leave me for. . . .

But by the time my son reached me, all feeling had miraculously returned to my arms and legs. I was so grateful that I went to Midnight Mass that night—although I must confess I left early after skipping ahead in the program and reading that we would all soon be asked to hold hands with the person sitting next to us, which in my case was the trailer dweller who sold Christmas trees in a nearby lot. But maybe I should've stayed.

Four months later, taking a short stroll, I suddenly became the scarecrow in *The Wizard of Oz*. My arms and legs went gimpy while the pain was like a cat-o'-nine-tails lashing me on the inside of my spine. You don't bluff Father Time or low-ball Uncle Mo. And me, in a heap on the sidewalk—that's called cheater's proof.

Rushed to the emergency room, I was scheduled to have what is called an MRI. Audio waves are trained through the water molecules in your body to create something like an enhanced x-ray. It sounded painless enough. Then I saw the man scheduled before me emerge from the MRI trailer. There was a noticeable shiver in his walk, and clumps of his hair had been sweat-moussed into a tangled frenzy, the way Jimmy Johnson's hair looked when they mussed it up at the Super Bowl, only he was smiling. This guy wasn't smiling.

"Take all your clothing off but your undershorts and put on this gown," the technician, a woman in her mid-twenties, instructed.

"Um, it seems I've left my shorts over in the other place," I told her, trying to sound dazed. She offered me another gown to wear backward, which I gallantly turned down—the last act of bravery I would muster for the next six hours.

Seeing the MRI machine for the first time could've added heart trouble to my growing list of maladies. A massive cylinder, with a conveyor belt leading to a small, tube like chamber cut through the center of it, took up half the trailer. It was like something out of *Star Trek*—or Forest Lawn.

● ●

Move Up If You Move Out

After a divorce, avoid the temptation to economize by moving into a cheap apartment. In fact, if it's at all possible, keep the same quality of housing you've been accustomed to or improve it a bit. A national survey found that men who remained homeowners, or who at least maintained an equivalent residence after the breakup, felt less stressed and depressed than recently divorced men who moved from a house to a rented apartment or to a lower-quality neighborhood.

"Okay, you're going to lie here, on the belt," the technician instructed, helping me up to the pyre, discreetly tending to her chemically treated hair. Gentle and reproving, she possessed the compassion found in people who work in stables—"We're gonna have to put Flicka down, son."

DEAD STILL

I was told to remain "dead still," not only an unfortunate choice of words but a daunting endeavor, since by now the hurt in my back was migrating from one area to another, whole fraternities of pain sensors swarming willy-nilly from kegger party to kegger party.

"You'll be inside for about 36 minutes," I was informed, and before I could object, she activated the conveyor belt. As I passed through the chamber arc, an ant riding on the tip of my nose, lifting his tiny head to cry for help, would've been decapitated. When the belt stopped, all of me was inside the chamber. Suddenly I was very, very big. The rounded surfaces were clad in that molded plastic used for the interior of airplanes, with miniature running lights producing the same, intimate lighting of a DC-10. But I wasn't flying. In fact, I wasn't going anywhere. With the ceiling so close to my face, I could see the pores in the nauseating plastic. My elbows touched the sides and the hardness invaded my senses. This was not a small reminder of what lies in the great beyond, I suddenly realized. This was a freaking dress rehearsal.

And then the pounding started. First, a single, shy knock, like someone at your bedroom door, afraid to come in and tell you something awful. It multiplied itself into a gurgling stream of moderate knocks and then it was quiet. A second later, the whole chamber exploded into a furious clatter, as if rescue workers with jackhammers were trying to pierce the shell. Panic began to suffocate me, and I had to talk myself down. I shut my eyes and dreamed of wide-open spaces. I tried to convince myself that it was Sheila E pounding out there and that she, too, forgot to wear undershorts. All I had to do was hang on for the time it takes to eulogize an unpopular dead relative. . . .

Afraid that they wouldn't hear me, I hollered over the

pneumatic pounding until suddenly the noises stopped and I felt the conveyor move.

"It's really okay," the sweet technician consoled me. "A third of the people who come in here can't go through with it."

Some hours later, I was shamed back into the MRI after being sedated to the point where if they had told me they planned to bury me alive, I would've dug the hole for them.

And even then I couldn't make it through the entire session without the reassuring touch of my wife, who reached into the chamber and held my big toe. That and singing the whole *Sergeant Pepper* album.

THE PHILADELPHIA COLLAR

But my humiliation was far from over. After the MRI, I was ordered to wear a device called a Philadelphia collar. The cruel irony in the name comes from the fact that wearing one gives you complete freedom from anything resembling self-esteem. This is a hideous prosthetic plastic cowl that forces your head back so that from afar, you look like a walking Pez dispenser. For the mechanically disinclined, the word "chin" is stenciled across the front of the cowl along with an arrow pointing at where yours should be.

Just about when I thought it couldn't get any worse, I got a phone call. I had been working on a project with two well-known married television stars. They wanted me to join them at their vacation home, pronto. When I told them about my back, they wouldn't take no for an answer. "We'll take care of it," they promised. "You won't have to lift a finger."

On the morning of the trip, a stretch limo pulled into my driveway. The chauffeur and a valet helped me into the back of the car, where the reigning Miss Iowa was waiting. She would be my traveling companion, in charge of pushing my wheelchair for the duration of the trip.

As we made our way through the Denver airport—the valet carrying my bags, Miss Iowa at the helm of my wheelchair, and I wearing the serf's collar of karmic shame that told the world I had done something truly stupid—we seemed to draw considerable attention. I felt sorry for Miss Iowa, a delightful and radiant young woman (who bore a resemblance to

Barbie's friend, Midge) consigned to wheeling around a falter-
ing, middle-aged geek wearing a flesh-colored potty seat
around his neck. I felt the eyes of strangers expressing a similar sentiment, so I apologized to her for it.

"Who gives a s—t what people think," Miss Iowa laughed,
steering my wheelchair into a squiggle.

These were wonderfully kind words. But they were the
words of youth, fortified by the luxury of supple bones and
sharp reflexes. It was all too clear that I had passed beyond the
high-stakes frolicking of Planet Reebok and the Just-Do-It generation. "A man's got to know his limitations," Dirty Harry, the
one-time mayor of sleepy Carmel, once said.

So be it. While I am not quite ready for softball and seniors
tennis, I have since learned to take life at a less calamitous clip,
to stop and watch the snow fall and, above all else, to don underwear when engaging in anything marginally risky.

—*Michael Angeli*

My Brothers, My Self

*We are side by side, racing over waves of red rock,
howling and snorting and cursing each other, riding
close together at death-daring speed, trying to knock
each other over. We're brothers.*

• • • • • • • • • • • • • • • • • •

IT IS A TREACHEROUS LANDSCAPE, as if sand dunes shifting and twisting had suddenly turned to rock. A solid stone sea
of swells, swales and cliffs. Plunging through it on our bikes,
we are laughing and elbowing each other even though a fall
would mean full-body bruises, deep scrapes, perhaps a broken
bone. It is a tradition, our tradition. An annual event just for us,
four brothers.

We are not boys anymore; we are men. A writer, a corporate headhunter, a gymnastics coach, a sculptor. Those are the men that everyone else knows. But they are not the men *we* know each other as. When we are together, we are brothers. We have the same blood, the same name.

Because we are no longer boys, we don't live together. We live in different cities in other states. We have houses and cars, lawns and plumbing problems. We have wives, ex-wives, children. We live our lives apart, writing stories or finding jobs for executives, teaching young girls to blithely somersault or working in bronze at three in the morning. These are the lives we have chosen.

We could do that. We grew up in the West, white, at the bottom of the middle class along with everyone else in our cow town. We were raised four houses from the prairie. We slept in bunkbeds. Red dirt blasting across the plains got into our teeth and our hair and our blood.

SIBLINGS FIRST

Riding reckless and mad through gullies, we are still husbands and fathers. But before that, we were brothers. Which means we know each other in certain ways better than our wives and children know us. We watched each other become men, helping and hindering in mischievous ways. We talked to each other about our wives, before we became their husbands.

Once we were athletes, all four of us, and we still are. We still tackle each other, still wrestle. We make jokes about guys we went to school with, football heroes and basketball stars, guys who've gone fat and flaccid. Physically and otherwise. We don't have mercy or empathy. We make jokes about a lot of things, but mostly about each other. We don't watch baseball. We don't golf.

When we left home, each in our turn, we discovered it was easy to forget we were brothers. We could become those other people. Brotherless people. This was years ago. To fix it, we decided to get together, just brothers, once a year, regardless. *Regardless.* That means wives and kids and jobs and bosses. That means money or time or distance. Even the hint of an excuse is drowned with derision. For this one three-day weekend, if you are a Jenkins brother, there is no good excuse on the face of the earth.

We meet at midnight on a Thursday in a strange city. Whooping and roughhousing, we throw our cowboy boots and bags in the trunk. Between sucker punches, we cinch four bicycles onto the roof rack. Then we drive through the night through the Rockies. We buy beer. We fight. Over conflicting myths of our own history. Over beautiful women we know and once knew. We fight over music: rock, country, reggae, alternative. A favorite tape goes out the window. Once, a shoe. We fart and shout. We wear sunglasses and snatch each other's baseball caps. The only thing we agree on is the Rolling

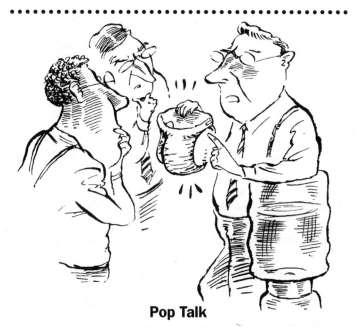

Pop Talk

Familiar scene? A bunch of guys standing around the office water cooler talking about . . . the Redskins? Steinbrenner? Would you believe diapers? According to research at Purdue University in West Lafayette, Indiana, one of the most talked about subjects on the job among first-time parents is babies, and that goes for dads and moms alike. But there is a gender difference. While women chew the fat about child-rearing stuff, "men tend to discuss consumer topics—where to get the best buy in diapers, a good deal on a stroller," says Douglas R. Powell, Ph.D., head of the Department of Child Development and Family Studies at Purdue University.

Stones. At the top of our lungs at 75 MPH over the passes in the dark.

We've had a long week doing all the things one must do to do nothing for three days, but we drive through the night, until we reach the desert and the dawn and can admit we're too exhausted to drive anymore. We pull into the sagebrush, take long stuporous leaks as the moon is paling, and fall into our sleeping bags.

STRIPPED BARE

Two hours later, somebody is laughing and pouring something on somebody's face. It's a bleary, bright morning, and we have escaped. We are in a different state. We have taken off our masks, stripped ourselves of the suits so carefully sewn. We are, again, just brothers.

We drive the last hour through the brown walls and up onto the mesa. We always go to the same hard rock place in the desert. It is the court of our competition. It doesn't matter what the world has done. If it is cold and snowy when we arrive, it is cold and snowy. If it is unbearably hot, so be it. It doesn't matter what you have done in the last year or what you have done to yourself. If you've grown weak, it is your problem.

As athletes, we are a mountaineer, a backpacker, a kick boxer, a cliff diver. But now we are only cyclists. The bicycle is the great leveler. No motor. No remote. Legs, lungs, balance. A song of motion and nothing more. We take the bicycles off the car, oil our chains and adjust our brakes and put water in our water bottles. And line up for the start.

We look over at each other. Then someone screams, the planet jolts and we are flying side by side across waves of red rock.

It is the same every year, a 13-mile loop through implausibly steep walls, deadly downhills, stretches of deep sand strewn with cactus. A perilous playground. None of us has ever made it unscathed. None of us ever will.

It is only a bicycle race through the desert. Four brothers no longer quite so young and hard doing something reserved for the young and hard, but we have rules.

The first is not even a rule, for it has always been so patently obvious that it has never been spoken: You can't quit.

You can't give up; you can't give in. One year it was 132 in the shade. One year our fingers were practically frostbitten.

The real first rule, indeed the only rule, is never to fall out of the saddle. The earth may buck and your steed may kick but you keep your ass in the saddle. It is a grueling three-hour rodeo through some of the cruelest country on Earth—a route that arcs along a high-wire rock rib a thousand feet above a river, then shoots down through a maze of roofless tunnels, then charges up walls so steep you are falling backward off your bicycle. But you keep your butt in the saddle and your feet on the pedals. Touch one foot and you not only get ridiculed, you get one point.

IF YOU HAVE TO ASK

The man who completes the course with the fewest points wins. Someone once asked me: What does he win? This person did not have a brother.

We all finish, sprinting, eight legs so fumbly and thick it is as if they're disconnected, four chests searing, four throats bellowing. Some of us lose and some win. We were not created equal. We were created brothers. Then it's into the nearby mining town for Mexican food and Mexican beer.

We ride hard all weekend. We dance and drink and close the cowboy bars. Sometimes when it looks like it might get out of hand, we are all four right there, standing beside each other, waiting for the first fist.

We sleep in the desert in the dirt every night. When Sunday evening comes and the sun is disappearing, tongueless and fightless and glue-eyed and hungover, we head home.

On the drive back the music is softer. We don't argue about it. We don't fight. We don't say we love each other. We don't have to. We just watch the highway roll out ahead and the moon slowly come up. We trade off driving and all of us sleep soundly. Soundly as boys.

—*Mark Jenkins*

The Father Business

No time to lament our own fathers' failings. We're all too busy learning how to be fathers ourselves.

● ● ● ● ● ● ● ● ● ● ● ● ● ● ● ● ● ● ●

I MUST BE THE ONLY MAN in my generation who had a father. For nearly a decade, men my age, Baby Boomers, have been creating a black hole in the past where Daddy used to be. The first I noticed was on August 21, 1984, when the *New York Times* announced that the American male was "troubled by the lack of a model for fatherhood." Said Joseph Pleck, director of the Male Role Program at the Center for Research on Women at Wellesley in Massachusetts: "In the 1950s, the big secret was that emotionally, Dad was not really part of the family." Shortly after, the complaint took a harsher turn in *New Age* magazine: "Chances are that if you are an adult between 20 and 55, your father was not a big part of your childhood, or big only in a negative way: remote, angry, repressed, vindictive. . . ." And that was just a start.

Lately, self-defined experts on this Distant Father syndrome have been using words like "abuse" and "oppression" to describe the typical Baby-Boom dad's child-rearing skills. The breadwinner of the '50s starved his children of vital emotional "nurture" simply by going to work in the morning, according to this theory. Robert Bly, in his book *Iron John,* likens commuting to a satanic crime: "When the son does not see his father's workplace, or what he produces . . . demons move into that empty place—demons of suspicion." In contrast, Bly lauds the era before 1900, when a boy "saw his father working at all times of the day and all seasons of the year." (He doesn't mention why they were so close: because entire families labored in the same factories, 14 hours a day, six days a week. How sweet.)

Back to reality: Why are we damning the fathers who provided for us? Why all this moaning about "hunger for the king in a time with no father," as Bly puts it?

I can see a certain reality in this attack on absent fathers. Many of our fathers died young (men still die younger than women); some were alcoholic, or broken in spirit. It's also true that half our parents' marriages went smash and that divorced fathers often cut off contact with their families. I remember the day my own father said, "I want to be free to live my new life" (which, to his credit, was more polite than "Let me the hell outta here!"), and how old I suddenly felt. Anyone who goes through such traumas has my sympathy.

SELF-SERVING DELUSION

Yet a big part of the Distant Father fad is based on an illusion—and not an innocent one. It's a self-serving fantasy, tricked out as a noble, progressive drama. In act one, men of my generation were childhood victims of powerful older men, asking to be loved, only to be rejected. In act two, to expiate our fathers' sins and heal ourselves, we became New Men, capable of working and loving in equal measure.

Funny, but that scenario doesn't account for all the facts—not the ones I saw, anyway. I don't know what you were doing in the late '60s, but I was driving my father out of the house with an electric guitar he bought me, smoking pot, making love with my girlfriend under his roof—hey, you think he felt jealous?—and telling him and his friends every chance I got that they were square, wrong and doomed, along with the rest of the "establishment." So was every self-respecting guy I knew. We were revolutionaries, man. Thus, I find it slightly weird when guys who sank their fangs into Daddy's hand complain that he didn't stroke them enough.

The second act of the Distant Father play doesn't stand scrutiny, either: We're not very different from the men who raised us, in terms of physical distance from our families. We want to be closer to our loved ones, but we're still the main providers, and therein is a bind. On average, men generate

• •

Shorts Story

It may just be time to throw away your old high-school gym trunks and get yourself a pair of larger, looser workout shorts. In a letter to the *New England Journal of Medicine,* a doctor described a patient who developed a mysterious swelling of his scrotum after doing stretching exercises. The doctor deduced that the man's gym shorts were too tight and prescribed a relaxed-fit pair.

nearly three-fourths of family incomes, and those earnings are reflected in hours on the job. Husbands usually work longer hours and travel farther to their jobs than wives do. That's why the average man with a working wife handles only 15 percent of the child care, according to the Census Bureau—a share that drops as his income rises. If he takes time for the family from his job, he risks putting a big dent in their standard of living. So he winds up trying to squeeze a size 12 life into a size 10 shoe. The day just isn't long enough to work and love equally.

You might say, "But our dads never even thought about this problem." I suggest you take a fresh look at *The Man in the Gray Flannel Suit*, Sloan Wilson's 1956 best-seller. Its hero, Tom Rath, knew he had to choose between ambition and his family, and when the moment came, he walked away from ambition, saying: "If I have to bury myself in a job every minute of my life, I don't see any point to it." It's significant that for most people, the man in the gray flannel suit is synonymous with abject conformity. That's a Freudian slip: We read even our fathers' rebellions against the system as selling out.

Like them, we've come up against a terrible conflict between work and love. Like them, we can't resign ourselves to it, or find a satisfying compromise—especially because the economy has tightened at the same time that our expectations of life have grown.

So we perform a magic trick. We acknowledge our conflict, and our pain, but we simultaneously project it into the past: That lonely guy in the mirror isn't us, it's Dad. He's the one who never had time both to win the bread and to break it with his loved ones, not us. Once again, we deny our fundamental likeness.

Unfortunately, no one can simultaneously deny himself and change himself. In refusing to identify with our fathers, we lose any hope of changing our own lives.

THE OEDIPUS IS US

There are striking parallels to our situation in the Oedipus story. A prophet foretold that the newborn Oedipus would kill his royal father, so the king set him out on the mountain to die. Saved by a shepherd, Oedipus grew up and set off to make his fortune. One day he killed a roadside bully, whom he later learned was his father. Stricken with remorse, Oedipus blinded himself and wandered the world, an outcast. Look: We too found our fathers blocking the path we wanted to take, and killed them in spirit. And now we are blind, to them and to ourselves.

Once we destroyed the breadwinner in our hearts and minds, we tried—unconsciously, yet eagerly—to bring him back. The same jobs and bosses we once revolted against suddenly became objects of slavish affection. "When you identify with your company's purpose," preached John Naisbitt in *Reinventing the Corporation,* "you find yourself doing your life's work instead of just doing time." Even former '60s radicals like Mark Gerzon celebrated the nurturing "frankness and openness" of the corporate culture, while *New Age* urged us to "do extraordinary work—and love it!" And so we became second-generation distant fathers, the revived image of our dads.

Sooner or later, we have to stop damning our fathers and repeating their mistakes. We have to change the system that wore them down and is wearing us down, too; find new ways of sharing work, income and love. That was the project we started in the '60s, then abandoned when we realized how hard it was going to be. But we can't blame our dads for that, or for refusing to help us try again. Not until we answer an urgent question: Why is it easier today for men to contact ancient tribal deities by beating on drums than to locate their fathers' phone numbers?

—Mark Hunter

A Stitch in Time

A wife cuts off her husband's penis. Most men cringe.
Most women find it unbelievably funny.

• • • • • • • • • • • • • • • • • •

DAVID BERMAN, MD., the gifted young surgeon who reattached the penis of a Virginia man after it was slashed off by his irate wife, reports he's heard from reporters "from all over the place. Japan. Italy. The British tabloids. Just about every radio station you can imagine."

Little wonder. This is a story that deals in some big-time universals: revenge and redemption, paranoia and (oh, God) pain. More than that, in the brutal sexual climate of the early '90s, it stands as a kind of Rorschach Test: Like the Amy Fisher case, what one sees in it depends almost entirely on the specifics of one's own history.

But first, the details. The guy in question, John Wayne Bobbitt, is a 26-year-old ex-Marine who was working as a bouncer; big on weight training, presumably someone who takes his body seriously, at 5-foot-11 and around 185 he bears a decided resemblance to Jean-Claude van Damme. The wife, Lorena, is a manicurist, 24 and darkly attractive.

Married four years and childless, they had been experiencing for some time, as the local Commonwealth's attorney delicately put it, "considerable domestic difficulty." Early on the morning of June 23, he returned to their Manassas apartment (near the legendary Civil War battlefield known as Bloody Manassas) with a friend after allegedly having been out drinking. While the friend went to sleep on the living room couch, the husband went to the bedroom where, according to the wife, he raped her and then fell into a sound sleep. She retreated to the kitchen, got a knife—reportedly one of those Ginsu knives they advertise on TV—and sliced off his penis.

"It was a real clean cut," notes surgeon Berman. "That thing must've been pretty damn sharp."

In any case, according to the same Commonwealth's attorney, this "awakened him quickly and abruptly."

GET RID OF THE EVIDENCE

Panic-stricken, apparently unaware she still held the penis, the wife fled the scene and drove off into the night; she would shortly hurl the evidence out the car window at an intersection, then, a while later, call the police from a pay phone and report its location. Meanwhile, the husband—incredibly enough, *not* panic-stricken—calmly woke the friend and had himself driven to the emergency room of Prince

William Hospital, arriving about 5:00 A.M. In fact, the details of his time in the emergency room might be the most amazing part of the entire story. "I couldn't believe it myself," says Dr. Berman, "so I checked it out with people who were there." It seems that, arriving in the emergency room holding a bloody sheet over his crotch, the guy was so nonchalant about his injury that, happening to find a friend waiting with minor injuries from a motorcycle mishap, "he starts listening to the guy ramble on about how he got all these cuts and bruises," says Dr. Berman. "And, obviously, the doctors and nurses have no idea it's even a serious injury. When the emergency room doctor walks in and sees the bloody sheet he assumes its a barroom injury and says, 'Lemme see your wrist.' He's just about blown away when he sees what the real problem is!"

The rest is medical history of sorts. Dr. Berman, new to the area, was reached at home by the urologist on duty and made it to the hospital about the same time as the penis, which had been recovered by police and packed in ice. Surgery began shortly after seven and lasted 9½ hours.

Though he'd never reattached a penis before, Dr. Berman, a master of understatement, insists the operation was fairly routine. "It's pretty much the same as a finger, just hooking up things correctly. It's precision work—you're using sutures the size of a hair, with tiny needles on them—but basically it's a technical skill. The thing to watch out for is that you don't impede flow-through. You're working with soft pipe, which can stretch or shrink, so it can bunch up.

"Since she'd left the stump of the penis, all we did was tie a piece of rubber around it to cut off bleeding and get to work."

The urethra, large enough not to require the use of the microscope, was reattached first, followed by the corporal artery, a tiny artery in the center of the penis. "If we had it to do over again, I wouldn't bother with the corporal artery, since it's not a major vessel," notes Dr. Berman, "but better to do too much than too little."

Next they sewed up the fascia, the heavy connective tissue around the penis; then two arteries, two nerves and a vein, and finally soft tissues and the skin.

JUST PINKED RIGHT UP

The doctors, Berman and the urologist who'd called him, weren't absolutely certain of the result until they removed the tourniquet; there was always the possibility of a leak, or worse. "But," notes Dr. Berman, "it just pinked right up fantastically."

Still, Dr. Berman remains somewhat guarded. "We can certainly say for sure he's not going to lose it now. It'll work; it's not gonna fall off or turn black. But when you repair a nerve, there can be scar tissue, so you might not get a full return of sensation. We won't know for sure about sexual function for a year." He pauses. "About a month after the incident, Bobbitt resumed light weight training, but I've asked him to hold off returning to his bouncer job for a while. He's really not ready yet for the trauma of a kick to the groin."

But fascinating as the medical details may be to the (pardon the expression) layperson, if this case proves one for the books, they will surely be psychology and sociology texts. Almost instantly, it took on a vast metaphorical significance and became a symbol of the remarkable depth of misunderstanding between the sexes. The hometown *Washington Post*, evidently sensing keener interest here than in, say, the concurrent budget deadlock in Congress, took after the story with a vengeance. On day two, there appeared a piece on the man- and woman-in-the-street reaction to the Manassas mauling. According to the paper that broke Watergate, the former

• •

One-Night Standards

Men and women have similar standards when choosing long-term partners. But when it comes to casual sex, researchers say men are like . . . well, animals. When psychologists at Arizona State University in Tempe questioned 327 college students about their criteria for marriage and steady dating, both men and women sought such qualities as intelligence, social status and attractiveness in a mate. But for one-night stands, women maintained their standards while men acted "like other mammals, undiscriminating," says researcher Douglas T. Kenrick, Ph.D. "Men are willing to go a lot lower in terms of intelligence, personality and the like."

gentler sex was not what you'd call real long on sympathy. "Every man's nightmare?" the *Post* quoted one woman as saying. "Every woman's is rape. So *c'est la vie,* buck. Now will all you guys stop raping us?" "Men have been doing this for years," added another. "It's time for people to be equal."

Not every woman reacted this strongly, but at breakfast tables everywhere, amazement seems to have been followed by laughter, at least from one side of the table. A woman friend tells me of the exceptionally high spirits among the females in her office that morning. The jokes on the excellent quality of cutlery these days and the kinds of commercials that might be shot to prove it; above all, thinking back on it, about what each of them would like to have done to this or that ex if only the occasion had arisen.

"This whole thing is just such an appealing power fantasy," as another woman friend put it. "Those odd appendages—and let's face it, they are funny-looking—just seem to mean so much to guys."

FAILURE TO COMMUNICATE

Odd appendages? Seem to mean so much? Talk about a failure to communicate! We are speaking here about a very, very close personal friend; someone with a personality all his own, not to mention a will and (in more cases than many of us will admit) a private nickname. Johnny. Big Red. Amarillo Slim. The Wanderer. Ivan (the Terrible).

Which is why men tended to react to the story by grabbing their crotches with a firm hand and keeping it there. The morning the story appeared in the *New York Times*—a sober, science-minded version, illustrated with a cross-section of a penis—I actually observed a half-dozen commuters reading

• •

Buy American

Consumer groups tested 110 brands of condoms from Portugal, Italy, the Netherlands, Brazil and Indonesia. Only 3 percent earned a "very good" mark. Over half of the brands were rated "very poor," and more than a third flunked a strength test.

the piece on a suburban train en route to Manhattan, each having unconsciously assumed precisely that position.

One doesn't have to talk to a psychologist to grasp what the prospect of a penis-less life would mean to most guys. But, earnest reporter that I am, I did anyway. Steven Manley, Ph.D., of the Dallas-based Male Health Center, confirms that "most men in such a situation would experience significant trauma. The penis is intimately bound up with identity." He adds that even altogether intact guys regularly ask about the matter of size.

How well we know. How many of us, in the privacy of our bedrooms, have taken out rulers and done the math? Which is to say that size *does* matter, at least psychologically. "I mean," as a friend of mine put it, "little's bad enough. But imagine trying to get through life with nothing."

CHILLING REACTION

Several I spoke to expressed consternation at the light-hearted female reaction to the incident. "What's chilling," a friend of mine said, "is how mean-spirited some of the comments have been. The hatred of men is so close to the surface."

Even some women agree. "There's this *Thelma and Louise*, let's-swig-a-little-tequila-and-shoot-'em-up kind of thing going," observes New Mexico sex therapist Carol Cassell, "and it says that anything a woman does to a man is legitimate. I mean, can you imagine if men turned that kind of anger on women? How would the media be treating this story if he'd cut out her clitoris?"

Then, too, she adds, "there's this notion that has been allowed to get around that somehow this is a case about a typical couple—that all men oppress all women and this is what can come of it. And that's just absurd."

As *Washington Post* columnist Tony Kornheiser sums it up, "Calling this a domestic difficulty is like saying Jeffrey Dahmer had an eating disorder."

Still, somehow, in the months after it broke and got filed away in the collective consciousness, the story had come to seem less shocking; a diverting skirmish in a war of misunderstanding and recrimination that has long since gotten out of hand. Now that there's a precedent, who will really be surprised to hear of such a thing happening again?

Not Dr. Berman, whose friends have taken to leaving messages on his answering machine for "the weenie doctor." Immediately after our conversation, he faxed a gag flyer a nurse had given him for a new insurance service for men. "Sign up now for our low-cost Penis Protection Plan. We'll register your penis and scrotum and tattoo them with their own unique registration numbers, insuring that in case of separation, you'll get a perfect match every time."

"It's pretty funny," observes the doctor. "Then, again, who knows what the future holds?"

—*Harry Stein*

Part 5

WOMEN AND SEX

Homework
for the Bedroom

Do sex therapists give homework? You bet they do!
Here are the favorite assignments of the Love Doctors.

• • • • • • • • • • • • • • • • • •

WHEN YOU HEAR THE PHRASE "sex therapy," what does it bring to mind? Erector sets for men? Scandinavian surrogates flashing a wry, knowing smile? Gene Wilder in *Everything You Ever Wanted to Know about Sex*, hiding out in a motel room with a sheep in a garter belt?

While the unusual is indeed a part of a sex therapist's practice, most of my patients are people who are probably very much like you—people who've had occasional problems with sex, who've sometimes felt bored with their partners, who've had affairs with unfortunate results. They're people who want help, but who are often afraid to ask for it. Seeking professional help with a sexual problem is part of our national ambivalence about these kinds of things: In our culture, virtually everything done with our pants down is supposed to be deeply rewarding. Yet, it's highly embarrassing to talk about.

Fortunately, there are also many things you and your partner can do to correct sexual difficulties and enhance your pleasure at home, and without a therapist's guidance. If sex is a problem, think of finding the solution as your homework. Home assignments may involve conceptualizing, talking, writing or touching. They may be done alone or as a couple. They may be designed to give people a chance to experiment or to practice techniques they've already learned. These experiments cannot be done wrong, since any "mistakes" you think you're making offer an opportunity for discussion and can lead to greater understanding.

But first, a prerequisite: be absolutely honest with yourself. Don't presume to know what's inside your partner's head. To accomplish that, learn to use the "I" statement. For example, "You don't love me" is mind-reading, while "I feel unloved" is at least an accurate assessment of your own feelings—though it may or may not have anything to do with your partner. Once both you and your partner have learned to focus on the problem without assessing blame, you're ready to start working on assignments that will help solve those problems. Here's a rundown of a few common ones.

PROBLEM: FLAGGING DESIRE

Assignment: Temporary ban on intercourse. Intercourse may be natural, but it's also the trickiest, most complex form of sexual expression—not least of all because so much of it is tied up in mechanical engineering. You're dealing with erection, lubrication, insertion and, typically, contraception—all at the same time—and you're doing it in the dark, because, let's face it, you can't really see what you're doing down there.

What to do? How about less of what isn't working. If you're unhappy with the quantity or quality of your sex life, make a rule: no intercourse for the next four to eight weeks.

You're probably saying, "Excuse me, Doc, but I'm reading this because I want *more* sex, not less."

But here's the thing: I'm not saying no sex, I'm saying no intercourse. No in-out, to use the technical term. That still leaves a vast array of erotic, sexual choices—from cuddling to cunnilingus—which I encourage couples to explore at their own pace. Eventually, partners often reveal to each other that they wish their relationship included more touching, kissing and caressing—much to the other's surprise. And because you're forbidden from having intercourse, activities like these are no longer "foreplay," a preliminary to the "real sex" that involves, after all, anxiety. They become, instead, ways to explore and enjoy each other's bodies, no more, no less. Often, when the ban ends, couples are ready to expand their repertoire.

PROBLEM: RAPID EJACULATION

Assignment: Sensate focus (touching exercises). *Sensate focus* is a general name for a group of exercises that focus on the experience of touch, as opposed to our thoughts about that touch. If you find yourself doing more thinking than feeling during sex, these exercises can be extremely helpful. Men troubled by rapid ejaculation (which used to be known as premature—a bit judgmental, don't you think?) are often tremendously concerned about being a "good lover." The problem isn't that they're not good, it's that they're worried they're not good. What to do? Tear down the goalposts. Sex isn't a game.

The key here is to get back to the enjoyment of touching, both yours and hers. Try this simple hand massage technique: For one minute, massage her left hand, in whatever way pleases you. Then switch to massaging her right hand, but this time attempting to please her as she gives you feedback. Then it is her turn to massage you in the same way. As she massages you, be certain to note all the aspects of the massage experience: texture, sight, smell and so on. Some men are very nervous when doing this assignment, especially in the role of receiving. But with practice, you'll learn to really relax and enjoy the massage.

PROBLEM: LACK OF INTIMACY AND LOSS OF DESIRE

Assignment: Breathing exercises. The only time we ever think about breathing is when we have trouble doing it. Yet, conscious breathing can be a powerful aid in sexual growth, and I make it a part of three closely related exercises.

1. Mirror breathing (for when couples aren't connecting sexually): Start by lying down close together, with the front of your body pressed against your partner's back. Lie quietly for a moment or two. Next, adjust your breathing so that it mirrors hers. Keep it in sync for 20 to 30 seconds. Then, as she slows down or speeds up her breathing, try to keep up. Repeat this several times, then reverse positions and start again. When discussing this later, many people report amazement that they were able to adjust to each other so subtly, and that they could feel so close without talking.

2. Slow breathing (for rapid ejaculation): This exercise involves deliberately slowing the breathing during sexual arousal. This is the opposite of our typical pattern, which is to breathe more quickly and shallowly as we get more excited. Slower breathing helps delay ejaculation by dissipating muscle tension and emotional anxiety. A similar exercise involves breathing deeply, as if into your pelvis. Imagine that as you inhale, the air flows not just to your lungs but all the way down to your pelvis, relaxing the pelvic muscles.

3. Coordinated breathing (for heightened sexual pleasure and increased intimacy): Finally, I recommend both male and female patients experiment with coordinated breathing. During regular intercourse, you exhale when you thrust toward your partner, inhale when you pull back. This heightens the physical sensations of sex and deepens the amount of stimulation we can tolerate before ejaculating. It also connects partners in a very special physical and emotional way.

PROBLEM: OBSESSIVE, UNWANTED THOUGHTS OR FUNCTIONAL DISTRESS, SUCH AS UNRELIABLE ERECTIONS

Assignment: Visualization. When top athletes are asked about their ability to connect a bat to a fastball or sink a 30-foot jump shot, they often credit their ability to visualize the feat beforehand. They see it happen before it actually does, and the physical follow-through becomes almost natural.

On the other hand, if the batter sees the ball coming and says, "No chance I'll ever be able to poke this out of the park," there's a good chance he won't. Imagine you're a guy having trouble with undependable erections. Your hard-on fluctuates like the price of gold: One minute it's up, the next it's down. Then, just before insertion, you say to yourself, "No chance I'll ever be able to keep this erection erect." No sooner said than done.

Try: Imagine, every single day, a satisfying sexual encounter. Imagine yourself and your partner undressing, getting aroused, having wonderful sex—intercourse, oral sex, whatever—for as long as you want, and only ejaculating when you're ready. See it happen. Some options to add, depending on your needs: Visualizing that you desire sex with a spouse or that you can easily ask for what you want in bed.

During all visualizations, your assignment is to be relaxed, playful and confident. After all, it's just you alone in the dark theater of your imagination. It's your movie. These mental run-throughs will not only give you confidence, they will also give your body permission to act the way you want it to.

PROBLEM: SOMETHING SO COMPLEX YOU CAN'T FIGURE IT OUT ON YOUR OWN

Assignment: Make an appointment with a professional. Sometimes a person or couple has a problem so big or complicated that they may need professional help. If, for exam-

• •

Squeeze Play

Impotence in some men may be treatable with simple exercises that strengthen the pelvic muscles, according to a study in Belgium. Seventy-eight men with a form of impotence caused by the inability to retain adequate blood levels in the penis were instructed to do a daily program of Kegels. These are simple exercises accomplished by squeezing the muscles of the rectum and those used in stopping the flow of urine. After four months, 42 percent of the subjects were able to satisfactorily maintain an erection.

ple, you and your partner find yourselves fighting all the time, if you want to get out of the relationship but can't or if being right is more important than solving the problem, then you probably need outside help. Seek the assistance of a marriage counselor, psychologist or sex therapist.

To find a good therapist, ask your physician, best friend or clergyman, or call the American Association of Sex Educators, Counselors and Therapists at (312) 644-0828. You may also find a specialist in sexuality in the yellow pages under Marriage Counselors or Psychologists.

—*Marty Klein, Ph.D.*

Going to the Sex Therapist

Does your marriage need major repairs or just a tune-up? Here are some facts every man should know about marriage counseling.

• • • • • • • • • • • • • • • • • • •

YOU'VE BEEN THERE. Over and over again. She tries to stir you up, and you try to calm her down; or she's having a bad day and trying to blame it on you; or it drives her nuts when you do things without her. Maybe at some point, the thought has gone through your head, "I can't take this anymore. One of us is crazy. I need somebody to talk some sense into that woman's head." Or another part of your brain says, "Maybe I need somebody to tell me what the hell *I'm* doing wrong." But then you don't do a thing about it. The storm passes over, and it's bearable for a while. So you forget about it. Until the next time.

I'm a psychiatrist, but I'm no different from any other guy. I have a hard time asking for help. Until a couple of years ago, I drove a secondhand 1971 Jaguar XJ6, a beautiful car in pale primrose yellow, but it would do weird things like jerk in and out of gear or lock up suddenly. My wife, who handles the money, kept telling me that it wasn't worth fixing, and we should get rid of it. My solution? I stopped telling her the weird things. Then one day, the transmission fell out on the expressway. When my wife came to rescue me, I admitted she'd been right all along. I'd never done that before. She was so excited, she found the money, and we bought a new car.

Most men are like me. We won't fix the car until the transmission falls out, and we won't go for therapy until the marriage is in very serious trouble. Some guys would rather change wives than go for advice. Others will have an affair with their secretary, yell at the kids, move to the guest room or storm out of the house so as not to end the marriage. But they still won't ask for help.

All this sounds crazy, but it's also understandable, considering that men are taught to solve problems by *winning*—not by admitting uncertainty or, worse, failure. Marriage therapy can seem like dangerous territory.

WHAT ARE WE AFRAID OF?

What are we so afraid of? We might say that we are afraid it will cost too much money, but often we know deep down that's just an avoidance ploy. What we really fear is acknowledging our helplessness and our failures. We fear humiliation, ridicule and shame about our most personal failings. We fear having our façade stripped away and our secrets unearthed. We fear having a therapist join forces with our partner against us.

Some of these fears are legitimate. There's no safety. The therapist is going to make us sit there and listen to a woman carrying on about us, even though we might prefer excluding all emotion and conducting the debate on a purely rational level. The therapist is going to expect us to explain ourselves, to take responsibility for our behavior and even to expose vulnerabilities and reveal secrets. We won't be able to do what we can do at home to stop the discussion or change the subject: We can't turn on the TV, walk out of the room or outshout her.

Sometimes at the therapist's office, we're on the woman's turf, playing by her rules and working toward her goals. It's unfamiliar ground for many men, but the wisest thing I've ever heard about marriage is simply that you can't always be right and be married at the same time.

Most of us know we're going to have to do some things differently if we expect to be happily married. We may even know what we don't do well and what needs changing. What we probably *don't* know, and can hope to learn from therapy, is why we're so scared. But only if we're willing to take some chances. To keep from exposing themselves, some men—even those who've agreed to counseling—will look for ways to wreck the therapy or to subvert it so that it will support their position, establish that they are right and don't have to change. It's perfectly possible to make it through marriage counseling without changing one iota. But, in my experience, men who succeed in preventing anyone from telling them that they are wrong will be rewarded with lifelong loneliness and unhappiness.

Winning isn't the point. Not in marriage. The point is to figure out what you're doing that doesn't work and to break down the barriers to change so that you can do things that will work better. It's a little like taking golf lessons: You start off knowing you're not Arnold Palmer and never will be, but you'd like to stay out of the rough more and get closer to the pin than you do now. The more things you learn that you're doing wrong, the less helpless you'll feel in achieving your goal.

There aren't all that many unsolvable marital problems. I rarely work with an established first marriage that ends in divorce unless somebody is screwing around and won't stop. I find that once two people get honest enough to understand each other, it is hard to pry them apart—even if they started therapy thinking they didn't like each other at all. Ultimately, though, it is not the therapist who makes a marriage work, it's the couple itself. Here are some things you should know before taking the first step.

When to go for marriage counseling. It's difficult to acknowledge that your marriage could use some help. But you don't have to wait until you're about to get divorced. You can go anytime you want some advice, even if, for the most part, your marriage is successful. And you also don't have to be married. Any relationship will do—unmarried, premarried, postmarried or polygamous. If the relationship really *is* on the verge of failure, the decision is a little easier. Anybody thinking or talking about divorce should go to couples therapy, even if the divorce is already under way or seems inevitable and desirable. Divorce is a disaster with consequences that reverberate for generations. Like amputation, it can save lives, but it leaves everyone's life diminished. The greatest horror of adversarial divorce is that some people can go all the way through it believing the legal gobbledygook and thinking the breakup was indeed irreversible, and the whole thing was their partner's fault. They think they married the wrong person. They don't learn anything that might help them do a better job next time.

What kind of therapist to go to. Seek out someone who is trained and experienced in dealing with relationship problems. Individual psychotherapists—as opposed to couples therapists—are trained to help their individual clients grow, but it is often by helping them to escape from imperfect relationships. If your marriage is fragile and valuable to you, and your partner won't go with you, go alone to a couples therapist. This person is trained to protect the relationship rather than sacrifice it as a quick fix for your pain. Some psychiatrists, an increasing number of psychologists, most social workers and members of the new profession of marriage and family therapists are trained to work with relationships. For a list of marriage therapists in your area and a free copy of a consumer's

• •

Shake and Rattle Poll

In case you were wondering whether porno films or vibrating sex toys were more arousing, *Archives of Sexual Behavior* reported on a study comparing the two. (Ah, science.) In the study, 34 men were exposed to both forms of stimulation. The guys were least aroused by using the vibrator, more aroused by the flick and downright feverish when given the vibrator while watching the movie. As for us, we found that reading *Archives of Sexual Behavior* was the least arousing.

guide to therapy, call the American Association for Marriage and Family Therapy at 1-800-374-2638.

What it will cost. Some therapists are booked months ahead and may charge as much as $200 an hour for their time. But plenty of well-seasoned and well-respected psychiatrists and psychologists and therapists charge half that or less. Your health insurance may pay part of the cost but is not likely to pay it all. Don't be discouraged if you have no insurance and not much money. Some private therapists and a lot of publicly funded clinics charge on a sliding scale. Whatever your circumstances, my advice is to put the money in perspective. If you can't afford therapy, you sure can't afford divorce. Which brings us to another point: A marriage in trouble is no place for well-intentioned amateurs. Don't turn to your buddies, your relatives or friendly strangers for advice on your marriage.

How to evaluate a therapist. Beware of anyone who makes you feel too comfortable. If the therapist is gentle and soothing and treats you as if you are an innocent victim and it's all your partner's fault, run for your life. If the therapist really pisses you off by trying to get you to take more than your share of responsibility for the mess, that's the one to hire. You're paying somebody to see you clearly, and to tell you, when necessary, what a jerk you're being and how you should shape up.

What you can expect. The therapist will spend the first session or so trying to define what the current problem is, what isn't working and where the impasse is. Then there will be a few sessions, sometimes together, sometimes separately, in which your family history will be explored so the therapist can examine why you have done what you've done—and why you have trouble doing what sensible people would do under the circumstances. As you progress, the therapist may assign tasks, not necessarily in the expectation that you will do them, but often just to find out which of you messes up the effort to make things work better and what the snag points are in your capacity for change.

The hard part. You will surely have to question most of the things you think you know about what it takes to be a man—traditional masculinity training is hard on men and hell on marriage. You will surely have to talk to your therapist and your partner about things you don't usually talk about, your insecurities in childhood, your losses and mourning, your vulnerabilities, maybe even your masturbatory fantasies.

An even harder part. Revealing your secrets. I have seen people who have kept secrets involving wealth, debt, extra children, prison records and even joblessness from their mates. People hide what they are ashamed of—even though in one way or another the shame or the feeling of inadequacy it produces is painfully evident to everyone. Infidelity is the biggie. Therapists differ about whether old, long-buried affairs need to be dug up and autopsied, but there's no question that current ones will need to be revealed—and the affair will usually have to end—before the magic of couples therapy can work. I often encourage a man who screws around to tell the whole truth to his wife and save the lies for the other women in his life. Who shares your secrets becomes your ally; who hears your lies becomes your adversary.

What's in it for you. Working on your marriage will change its course, nearly always for the better. Therapy should also make you more loving and more lovable, more communicative, more fun, more secure, more confident and more free. You'll learn where you learned to feel the things you feel that hurt you, and where you learned to do the things you do that don't work. Marriage therapy can get you past your mourning for past relationships, your pain over past hurts, your shame about your inadequacies, your guilt about your betrayals, your anxiety about whether anyone could love you. Once you get into it, it should feel good.

Remember, it's your marriage, perhaps the most important investment of your life. Value it and pamper it before the transmission falls out and you have to junk it.

—*Frank Pittman, M.D.*

Love Potions and Spells

Want to become a sex object? Get right in line.
Romance takes some luck, some skill and some
secrets. Here are the secrets.

●●●●●●●●●●●●●●●●●●●

You'd THINK, AFTER ALL the careful scrutiny men have given to sex objects, we'd have a better idea how to be one ourselves. Most of us are so convinced that we ought to be the sex subject of a sex object that we never give women the chance to objectify us.

Besides, sometimes our goals are not so lofty. Sometimes all we want is to drive women insane with desire. Is that so much to ask? Not at all. The trick is to make a woman stop seeing you as a thinking, feeling, complex person with hopes and dreams and visions, and start seeing you as a simple tool for doing a simple job. Objectification is a goal that's within the reach of every man. All you have to do is grab for it. Here are the four paths.

1. Don't try so hard. Take a friend of ours, Mr. F. He recently moved to a swank southern metropolis. On the way he drifted through a half-dozen eastern cities, pausing once in New York City—where he enjoyed, he said, "a certain kind of relationship" with a beautiful artist in a car parked in an alley—and once in Baltimore, where he was found in a cocktail lounge unable to handle his alcohol, because the two women between whom he was sandwiched wouldn't take his hands from their laps. When he arrived in Dixieville, he was, he said, "automatically given women when I crossed the city line." After a monumental sexual olympiad, he finally had to take a breather, because he clocked himself in the noggin on a side table while performing some libidinal legerdemain. "Now I'm thinking about buying a house," he said when he came to, "and filling it with a wife and kids." Alas, he added, "There are just so many women to choose from."

All women love Mr. F., and, as a consequence, he is having sex for all the rest of us. Why? Mr. F. understands that women are immensely interested in men who are pleasant, charming, witty and, above all, pleased to be in their company without any expectations. "I guess sex just never crosses my mind," Mr. F. said, "but it's nice when it crosses theirs." By not making women into sex objects, Mr. F. allows them the liberty of making him into one, and he hates to disappoint.

So what can we learn from Mr. F.?

You usually get more than you need if you don't ask for anything at all.

2. Give it everything you've got. Some men are more action-oriented than Mr. F., and there are some women who can only be found—much less wooed—with an all-out storming of the gates. A man I know, whom I shall call Mr. Coyote, is a master of blitzkrieg lovecraft. Coyote sees an attractive woman, and he immediately thinks Road Runner. All of a sudden, huge, cast-iron safes full of romance are tumbling out of the sky, there are explosions everywhere, and, without being asked to, he's running off the edges of cliffs into thin air.

Sometimes a woman sees this sort of behavior, says, "What the hell," and is swept up into some pyrotechnic scene in which her previously stark, unadorned life suddenly looks like a Jimi Hendrix poster. Then she finds herself doing all the things she swore she'd never do, including the Polaroid thing. Two weeks or two months later, she's saying, "Beep, beep," and vanishing into the landscape in a cloud of dust.

Mr. Coyote has winter wives and summer brides, but no relationship that stretches across more than two major holidays, for nothing can stand up to such an acute level of stress. But Coyote is 100 percent sex object and just glad to be out there.

There is something to be learned here, by the rocket's red glare: If you're going to be a wolf, leave the sheep's clothing at home. There's no sense hoping some woman is going to grab you by the lapels of your sensitivity suit and rip your clothes off. Go naked.

3. Listen a little, love a lot. Mr. Bill isn't the most handsome guy, and while he can outwit his dinner, he's not a genius by any stretch. As a teenager, he was foiled on dates, just like the rest of us. Couldn't get to first base. But in college, he learned a valuable lesson: women, as dates, liked men who liked women, as a movement. So he would take his dates to feminist lectures and women's issues rallies, raising their consciousness with the warm, cozy fires of the sexual revolution crackling in the background. Women loved it.

Mr. Bill is now a well-known man, and some women—total strangers, mind you—dream about him. Nasty stuff, too. To them, he is a dreamboat, a sex object.

Lessons? Sometimes, women like the idea of two equal souls slapping bellies in the night. That's one. And two: Good conversation can have a certain intimation of carnality.

4. Find a principal who's a good teacher. Contentious from birth, men strive to vanquish one another, or, failing that, to find a quiet corner where other men will leave them alone. In commerce, the victors are obvious, since the spoils of war—homes, cars, trophy wives—are quite visible. But when it comes to emotional gamesmanship, it's women who are the referees, the ones who decide who's a winner and who's a loser. That's why some men need a woman who can teach them the rules of the game.

Take, for instance, a stockbroker whom I'll call Q. He was financially successful, reasonably handsome, yet filled with self-doubt. He would ask his friends hideous questions: "Do I seem stupid?" or "What can I talk about to make me seem important?" His friends were mortified for him, and so, of course, were most of the women he dated, since he sought from them some creepy affirmation. Then, one day, he met a woman whom he thought unattainable—smart, confident and scenic. Remarkably, and to the immense confusion of his friends, the beauty liked Q. They married and Q settled down with his wife. But not only that. There was another party to the relationship: his new, confident, interesting, concerned self.

His friends watched this transformation in fear, but the marriage was apparently sound. Eventually, several of Q's friends collared him and asked him how he had done it. "I didn't," Q said, "she did. She would pick a fight with me whenever I asked those stupid questions, the ones that made me look so lame. The fight would be about something else, something that didn't have anything to do with my doubts. Then she'd let me win the argument."

Q's wife refused to let him slip into full-nelson dorkiness. In his new, more masculine wardrobe, he's her sex object.

The lesson of Q: It's one thing to be a man among men. It's another to be a man among women.

Four paths, one goal: to get what you want out of a bedroom, other than a good night's sleep. Remember, we're surrounded by women, the very people who can cause us the greatest joy and most profound anguish. Here's the key: It's the joy part you want.

—Roger McElvey

Dream Loving

Been having some strange sex dreams lately? Join the club. Here are some clues to what they mean.

• • • • • • • • • • • • • • • • • • •

IF YOU DREAM THAT YOU'RE having sex with the butcher's wife, or the butcher or even the butcher's dog, don't panic. Although few of us will admit it, most of us have had the same or similar dreams, too. Strange sex dreams, even those that may seem disturbingly perverse by daylight, are an almost universal human experience.

The late Alfred Kinsey, D.Sc., found that nearly all men had sex dreams, often so torrid they resulted in orgasm. Interestingly enough, Dr. Kinsey also found that the better educated his subjects were, the more often they had sexy dreams. For instance, adolescent boys who later went on to college had nocturnal emissions triggered by sex dreams *seven times* more frequently than boys who never made it beyond grade school. Dr. Kinsey attributed this difference to the greater imaginative capacities of the brighter boys. Feel free, in other words, to consider your next steamy dream as proof of your superior intelligence. Don't forget, though, that even animals appear to have sex dreams. There have been some reports of sex

WORKING OUT THE KINKS

The experts assure us that dream behavior, even stuff that would get you locked up in real life, is a harmless venting of our inner needs and frustrations. Following are their interpretations of the most frequent sex dreams.

Cheating dreams. Dreams that involve a woman other than your wife or steady girlfriend are no cause for guilt. In fact, they may help keep you in line in real life, says Robert Hicks, Ph.D., a psychology professor at San Jose State University in California who studies dreams. You may have remembered only the sexual parts of the dream, but it's not unlikely that you dreamed about the drawbacks—being caught, losing your family—later on in the night. "These dreams help us explore the consequences without having to make the mistakes," says Dr. Hicks.

Dreams about sex with an unattractive person. "This is a common dream for younger men," says Dr. Hicks. "It's a way of exploring what the qualities of a proper mate are and whether you can relate to someone who looks unappealing." These dreams usually fade as we get older and realize that not all our partners will look like Michelle Pfeiffer.

dreams in a cat (with ejaculation), a shrew (with a teeny erection) and dogs.

And remember, you're not the only one in your bed dreaming about wild sex. Your wife is doing some steamy dreaming, too, maybe even more than you are. In fact, sexual dreaming in men peaks while they're still in their late teens or twenties, but women have the most sexual dreams in their forties. Yet the visions that appear to your partner at night may be very different from your own. In one study of 100 male and 100 female college students, women were more likely to dream about kissing and petting, men more likely to dream of intercourse. And while the men seemed quite happy dreaming about strangers, women's dream lovers were more likely to be someone they actually knew.

Homosexual dreams. Remember that sexual encounters in dreams are often metaphors for unrelated feelings. If you've had recent difficulty in a relationship with a woman, for example, a homosexual dream may actually be a way of comforting yourself. "You, as a man, understand how guys think," suggests Robert L. Van de Castle, Ph.D., a behavioral psychologist and dream expert at the University of Virginia in Charlottesville. "They're not this mysterious opposite sex that's so hard to figure out."

Frustration dreams. Dreams in which sex is imminent but you never quite close the deal are often about other frustrating aspects of your life, says Dr. Hicks. Anxieties about not getting a new work project off the ground can manifest themselves this way.

Incestuous dreams. Perhaps the most disturbing dreams of all, they don't represent some deep-seated perversion, Dr. Van de Castle explains. "These dreams can occur when we're not doing well in our dating or our relationships." By seeking out a family member, we're finding comfort in someone with whom there's no fear of rejection. The dream may be suggesting that we have to try harder to make our relationships work.

Women, of course, don't leave incriminating evidence that they've had a sex dream; we sometimes do. Wet dreams, or nocturnal emissions, tend to begin a year or so after a young boy reaches adolescence and reach their greatest frequency during the teens and early twenties. Still, Dr. Kinsey found a huge variation: About 17 percent of boys never have wet dreams at all, while others have them so frequently it becomes a laundry problem.

If this all seems like an awful lot of energy to expend while we're supposed to be catching up on our sleep, consider that these x-rated little dreams are actually good for us. Sex dreams are a way of discharging physical urges in a safe, harmless way. And experts say that if some of these nocturnal fantasies are disturbing to our waking sense of propriety, it's best not to get too worked up about it. "It's really not that unusual for a heterosexual man to have an occasional homosexual dream," says Robert L. Van de Castle, Ph.D., a behavioral psychologist and dream expert at the University of Virginia in Charlottesville.

EVERYTHING IS SEX

To hear Freud tell it, of course, almost *everything* in dreams—and in life—is sexual. In his view, dreams are the fulfillment of some repressed infantile wish—nearly always a sexual one. Since these wishes are usually unacceptable to the conscious mind, the theory goes, the unconscious mind expresses them in dreams in disguised, symbolic form. In Freudian dream interpretation, every image that's a receptacle (boxes, bowls, houses) or enclosing (rooms, tunnels) is taken to be a symbol representing the vagina. So are mouths, ears and eyes. Everything that's oblong or suggests penetration (sticks, knives, umbrellas, pencils, cigars), along with hands and feet, represents the penis. Walking up and down stairs or ladders suggests intercourse (bouncing up and down—get it?).

The trouble is, not all sex dreams are about boxes or umbrellas—sometimes they're as blatantly, unashamedly sexual as a naked breast. This poses a real problem for Freudians, who are forced to argue that this sort of dream conceals a still deeper, more taboo sexual urge. But "this argument that nothing is ever what it appears to be is very unconvincing to me," says Dr. Van de Castle. "If, according to

• •

I Dream of Jeannie, and Vice Versa

Women daydream about sex, just as you do, Bubba. And those women who often daydream about sex have more positive attitudes about sex and more orgasms, and are more sexually satisfied, than women who daydream less often, according to a recent survey of 117 women. Those who had sex 50 times or more a year had more sexual daydreams than women who had sex fewer than 50 times a year. The frequent daydreamers also reported more closeness with their partners that was nonsexual.

Freud, all weapons and tools are symbols standing for the penis, then what does it mean when one dreams about a penis? Does it mean that the person is really dreaming about a gun or a hammer?"

Anyway, all their arcane arguments aside, psychologists and dream experts generally agree on one thing: If you have a torrid sex dream, regardless of who or what it was about, don't get worked up over it. Enjoy the free entertainment.

—Stefan Bechtel

Sexual Signals

Women seem to speak their own very special, very secret language. Here's a pocket translator to keep you out of trouble.

● ● ● ● ● ● ● ● ● ● ● ● ● ● ● ● ● ● ●

Why is it that the nation that invented *Classics Illustrated* and *Monarch Notes* hasn't yet figured out a way for men to get a read on women? Wouldn't it be easier if women would just come out and tell you, "Leave me alone, you cretin," or "Why don't you stop by to see my etchings?" Well, they often do. The problem is that for women, actions speak louder than words. Unfortunately, when it comes to gestures, women are usually talking in a language men don't understand. When a woman thinks she is telling you, in plain English, to leave her alone, you're hearing love-polka lyrics in Slavic and coming on like gangbusters.

What accounts for this gross level of misunderstanding? Body language. Body language is the Berlitz of intentions. It reveals everything you need to know about a woman at a glance. Master it and you'll be able to find your way to first base no matter where you roam.

What you need to know: First of all, if body language is

your lingo, make sure she's talking to you before you try to answer her in her native tongue. For example, you are sitting next to a colleague in a board meeting, and she inadvertently brushes her hair from her eyes. Is she saying, "I need sex now!" or is she saying, "Damn hair. Wish it wouldn't fall in my eyes"? Since there's no sure indicator that a woman is open to an advance, you need to look for a combination of signals, says Jonathan Kramer, Ph.D., author of *Why Men Don't Get Enough Sex and Women Don't Get Enough Love*. "If she's touching your arm during a conversation, don't just take it as sexual because you want it to be sexual." Jump to conclusions and next thing you know, whack! Another slap in the face, another day in sexual-harassment court, another day in the unemployment office.

Once you're absolutely certain she's trying to say something to you, you can begin to try to understand what it is she's saying. Here, to help, is a phrase book for tourists in Woman-World, where every small thing counts and where sensitivity is the pocket change of basic thought.

THE EYES HAVE IT

Eye contact. It's generally a good sign if a woman actually looks at you when she speaks—much better than if she stares unblinkingly at her fingernails or her shoes and mumbles. Two people conversing look at each other about 60 per-

· ·

Flirtation Device

A woman smiles at you. Is she interested, or is it a cover for what she's really thinking—"Get out of my face, Bucko"? According to one study, the proof of a genuine smile isn't in the lips but in the eyes. Researchers showed videotapes of smiling women to a group of college students and asked them to judge whether the smiles were real or phony. The students guessed right up to 74 percent of the time, and those who judged a smile by watching the eyes were more accurate guessers. Genuine smiles trigger a slight closing of the eyes and a wrinkling of the skin around them; fake ones tend to last longer and have little effect on the eyes.

cent of the time, according to Michael Argyle in his book *Bodily Communication*. So if you catch her looking at you more than 60 percent, chances are she's more interested in you than in what you're saying.

Smiles. A broad smile is a sign of real enjoyment. But be on the lookout for a smile that shows only the upper teeth. It's a polite smile—or one that shows a woman is feeling uncomfortable.

Movement. A woman who shifts her body around as she speaks to you may be sending a message: "Movement attracts attention," says Colleen, a 35-year-old legislative assistant. "If I'm adjusting my posture, it means I'm attracted." She might, she says, even roll her hips a little if she's talking to you.

Leaning toward you. Leaning in, tilting her head to one side, speaking in a softer voice: According to experts, these may all indicate interest.

Giggling. Laughing in a charming, feminine way is a positive. On the other hand, if she lets out a guffaw, it probably means she just wants to be considered one of the guys.

Flushed face. That's a good sign, because your blood flow increases when you're attracted to someone. "Her pupils may dilate, too," says Judee Burgoon, Ph.D., professor of communication at the University of Arizona in Tucson. But, she cautions, pupils also dilate when you're hungry, so make sure she's thinking beefcake and not hamburger.

Touching. Julius Fast, author of *Body Language*, says women sometimes touch men during conversation. Laying a hand on a shoulder or a forearm or playing with a tie—all are signs of flirtatiousness.

Touching herself. If she's flipping her hair, fixing her clothes, playing with jewelry—those are all positive signs. "She may affect a gesture in which one hand touches her breast in a near caress. She may stroke her thighs as she talks," says Fast. That's the basic lexicon of body talk.

QUIZ YOUR NEW KNOWLEDGE

Pop quiz: Let's just see how well you have it all down. If a woman you're talking to is staring at her wristwatch with a frozen smile plastered across her face and sitting as if she's dreaming of Preparation H, is she . . .

> **a.** Struggling to hide her burning desire for you?
>
> **b.** Waiting for a bus?
>
> **c.** Wishing you were choking on your lunch in another country?

The correct answer: C.

Let's try again. Suppose you walk up to a woman, say, "Hiya, howya doin?" and she says, "Pretty good," while staring into your eyes and rolling her hips. She giggles softly, her face flushed with passion, while she caresses a breast with one hand and rubs her thigh with the other. Does this mean . . .

> **a.** She's pleased to meet you?
>
> **b.** She's covered with poison ivy?
>
> **c.** She might be open to a conversation, but nothing in this life is certain?

Answer: C again. She may be interested in you, but you still never know for sure. If you're right, you go straight to bed. If you're wrong, straight to jail. It's a tough call. No wonder men love to watch.

The problem is, just knowing these clues can't guarantee you'll understand what's being said. You need more signals (although the breast caress and thigh rub bit is a pretty strong hint). The rule of thumb: Where she is when she's talking body talk is as important as what she's saying.

Here, then, is the second part of our lesson, a field guide to the natural behavior of the female of our species, no matter where she's spotted.

Bars. In a bar, you're working on the relatively safe assumption that a lot of the women there have come to meet men. Dr. Burgoon suggests you watch for positive signs like lots of smiling, straightening of clothing, twisting of hair around fingers. But don't necessarily expect her to char your eye sockets with a blazing stare; she's got her pride, you know.

Parties. The party scene differs from the bar scene in

that you can't assume the women there are looking to meet someone. Plus, it's likely you'll have mutual friends there, so making a move when it's not your turn can look especially bad. Look for the same clues you might see at a bar, only more so. Since it's a social event, not a "scene," there's more time to speak to someone after your initial meeting. That means there's more time for a woman to make her feelings clear. If your conversation is going smoothly, Dr. Burgoon suggests you watch to see if she is mirroring your moves. Consider it a good sign if she keeps her body directly in front of you when you move, or if she tilts her head in the same way you do. "It's like dancing," Dr. Burgoon says.

The gym. Oh, the joys of physical fitness—unless you're a woman who doesn't want to be picked up. How will you know her? By her headphones, says Amanda Benedict, an aerobics instructor at Fitness Advantage Health Club in San Diego. Women who don't want to be approached have their phones on snugly and keep their eyes focused on the floor, the machine or the mirror straight in front of them. On the other hand, if she *is* interested, she'll watch you work out. Another positive: if she looks at you, looks away and then takes off those blasted headphones. Also, be helpful to a woman who's acting helpless. Her question about how to use a machine could easily be a come-on.

The beach. Here, the same signals that mean "talk to me" elsewhere don't always apply. "She may be looking for a friend and scanning the beach when her eyes meet yours," says clinical psychologist Andrea Johnston, Ph.D. She might be fixing her hair, because it got caught in her suit. That doesn't necessarily mean she wants you to come over. Still, there are clues: Minnie, a 24-year-old secretary, says a guy can assume a woman is looking to meet someone on the beach if her hair is in place and isn't wet. Another obvious beach blanket bingo ploy: She'll hold her stomach in. (I guess sometimes women and men do behave alike.) You can easily spot the woman who wants to be left alone—she's the one wearing sunglasses, lying on her stomach and reading a book.

The office. There's a very delicate line between asking a colleague out to lunch and sexual harassment. If you're talking with a co-worker and it's not entirely business, make sure all the signs are there. Look not only for casual touches on the sleeve or shoulder, but for intimacy or sexual innuendo in the conversation as well. "Better to err on the side of not being too forward," says Dr. Johnston.

The most important thing in all this is not to take any one cue as definitive. The eyes, the smile, the posture all work as a system. But it's a system worthy of study. Some experts claim that 90 percent of our communication is nonverbal, which is to say that if men spent more time watching what women do with their bodies, instead of just watching their bodies, we could declare a truce in the war of the sexes.

—*Eilene Zimmerman*

Part 6

DISEASE-FREE LIVING

Don't Ignore
These Symptoms

*You are the first person to interpret your symptoms.
Better have a look at these 15 problems that could
be serious.*

• • • • • • • • • • • • • • • • • • •

MY FRIEND WAS CONVINCED he had a brain tumor. Ringing in the ears, head pain, hearing loss—all the signs were there. But rather than see a doctor and receive confirmation of his impending demise, he suffered through, even scratching out a will. Finally, the discomfort became too much. He broke down and confessed his ailment to his family doctor, who then examined the man and made his diagnostic pronouncement: earwax. Lots of it.

Like most men, my friend jumped to a conclusion and suffered the consequences. While women, when faced with something painful or unexplainable, will actively seek to dispense with both pain and apprehension by going to a doctor, most men prefer to come up with an answer on their own. And like my friend, we often assume the worst, even though in many cases severe pain has an innocuous cause.

Sometimes, however, the situation is reversed, and even minor pain can be a sign of a serious problem. For example, "I can't tell you how many people think they have heartburn when they're really having a heart attack," says Jorge Herrera, M.D., a spokesman for the American Gastroenterological Association. With that in mind, we've looked into a wide range of symptoms and what might be causing them, with an eye on the bottom-line question: When do I see a doctor? Herewith, a guide.

1. Afternoon slump. Even hard-charging men find that mental and physical energy flags between 1:00 and 3:00 P.M., thanks to sleep-wake patterns governed by our biological clocks. If, however, you find that your afternoon slump hits you extremely hard no matter how early you go to bed, you may have a sleep disorder that's preventing you from getting enough rest.

A likely suspect is sleep apnea, in which nighttime breathing stops periodically for ten seconds or more, producing a gasping reflex that partially awakens you. This is particularly common in snorers.

When to see a doctor: Two or more weeks of unaccountably heavy slumps often lasting well into the afternoon or evening. You may have a sleep disorder that's costing you more than shut-eye: People with chronic sleep apnea run an increased risk of high blood pressure.

2. Arm pain. When arm pain feels different from run-of-the-mill achiness, you need to pay attention to where and how it's hitting. In particular, take seriously any sudden, strong pain in the upper arm. Because it's so well-muscled (at least that's what we tell ourselves), the upper arm isn't inclined to hurt badly unless something's wrong elsewhere.

If pain sneaks up gradually and lingers, it's possible you

have a broken bone; fractures sometimes don't make themselves known for days.

When to see a doctor: Upper arm pain is accompanied by chest pain, nausea or shortness of breath. These are the classic symptoms of a heart attack, and you need immediate attention. See your physician, too, if your arm hurts for more than two days; the pain gets worse with work or exercise; you lose feeling; you can't move or straighten the arm or the arm becomes deformed or swollen. Broken bones or inflamed tendons are a likely cause and should receive a physician's attention.

3. Bad breath. Sure, it might be that anchovy and garlic pizza you polished off last night, but more likely your malodorous exhalations are a product of bacteria. And getting rid of it isn't just a dainty matter of social correctness. Chronic bad breath more often than not indicates *gingivitis* (gum inflammation) or *periodontitis,* an even more damaging gum disease, both caused by bacterial buildup on teeth and gums. One obvious cause of bad breath is inadequate brushing or flossing. (Hint: Do a once-over brush of your tongue and the inside of your cheeks, which harbor the same bugs as your teeth.) Another cause may be dry mouth, since a lack of saliva means a lack of the bacteria-killing enzymes it contains. It's normal to have a dry mouth in the morning (blaming your enzymes is a handy excuse to drop on an offended bedmate), but sinus-drying medications like antihistamines and certain antidepressants can also parch the mouth.

When to see a doctor: Head for the dentist if regular floss-

● ●

Binding Resolution

The next time you have the runs, run to your kitchen and blend up a banana-orange punch. When you have diarrhea, your first order of business—well, maybe your second—should be to replenish lost fluids and important nutrients. From this standpoint, orange juice has it all—water, vitamins, minerals and calories. A nice ripe banana makes it even better, adding needed potassium, which diarrhea depletes from the body. Also, bananas contain pectin, which absorbs water like a sponge, helping to put a stop to the problem.

ing along with a thorough brushing of the teeth and tongue fail to eliminate the odor; it's likely you'll need a cleaning. If a foul odor is accompanied by bleeding, swelling or pain in your mouth or throat, you may have gum disease; consider seeing a periodontist.

4. Body ache. You've been doing some heavy lifting or you recently challenged your 19-year-old cousin to a pickup game. Overdo it and you're bound to be sore the next day—or even two or three days later. Muscle soreness may not hit you right away, and after a body-jarring fall or accident, it may grow progressively worse for a few days before it gets better. The best defense against soreness is to take over-the-counter, anti-inflammatory pain relievers like aspirin or ibuprofen—and take it easy for a couple of days.

When to see a doctor: Any unexplained body ache may signal a viral infection. Ditto for achiness that continues for more than five days or continues to get worse. Also, keep an eye out for an accompanying rash that could signal Lyme disease.

5. Clicking jaw. A noise is often caused when tired or overworked muscles fail to pull the jaw bone through its motions evenly, which is common on an occasional basis and nothing to worry about.

Sometimes, however, jaw clicking is caused when muscles and ligaments that support the joint are overly stretched and chronically out of alignment, making the bones of the jaw grind together all the time—a condition called temporomandibular joint disorder (TMD). In some cases, it can lead to a lockup of the jaw and headaches, as well as pain in the jaw and neck.

When to see a doctor: Visit your dentist if clicking or tooth grinding is chronic or accompanied by pain, which could indicate TMD. Nine out of ten people whose jaws click regularly also clench and grind their teeth in their sleep, a habit that can erode chewing surfaces and cause the jaw to deteriorate.

6. Earache. Contrary to popular opinion, most earaches are not instigated by neighborhood teens blasting heavy-metal music by groups with names like Horrible Throbbing Death. Actually, they're generally precipitated by viruses and bacteria taking root in the ear where they form pus that pushes painfully against the eardrum. To relieve ear problems, first try clearing the eustachian tubes by swallowing, chewing, yawning or using an over-the-counter decongestant spray like Neo-Synephrine. Take an analgesic like acetaminophen or ibuprofen to kill the pain, and prop yourself up in bed to reduce ear congestion.

When to see a doctor: Ear pain lasting more than a week is a sign of infection; the danger is that, if left untreated, the infection can burst the eardrum. Your doctor can prescribe an antibiotic to quell the problem.

7. Ringing in the ears. It's only a problem if it's persistent. Maybe you've been standing too close to those incoming commuter trains. Such prolonged exposure can cause the nerve endings of the inner ear to wear out and send phantom signals to the brain. For starters, avoid cigarettes, caffeine and salt, which can stimulate or swell hearing mechanisms, aggravating the problem.

When to see a doctor: Ringing is accompanied by dizziness or pain. You may also be suffering from a bacterial infection, fluid in the middle ear, a hole in the eardrum or a big plug of wax. Less likely, but possible, are Ménière's disease, a mysterious ailment that attacks the inner ear, or a tumor on the auditory nerve of the inner ear.

8. Headache. You know from experience that headaches generally mean nothing more than that you've had a bad day. But persistent headaches can also be a sign of a potentially hazardous health problem.

Then there are cluster headaches, attacks that predominantly affect men and are excruciating enough to be taken seriously in and of themselves. Imagine badgers are trying to gnaw out of your brain via your eye socket, and you'll understand their power. Following are some quick headache fixes.

• •

Heavy Metal Vitamin

If you listen to loud rock 'n' roll or like to shoot guns, ear plugs and vitamin B_{12} may be in order. Tinnitus, an ear disorder that causes a constant buzzing or ringing in the ears, has been linked to a vitamin B_{12} deficiency, according to a study of soldiers in Israel. Treatment with B_{12} shots improved tinnitus symptoms in some patients.

- When your head hurts, try exercising. You may not feel like working out, but exercise relieves stress and can trigger production of natural painkillers called endorphins.

- Get the blood flowing with a heating pad. Warming the neck and shoulders for 15 to 20 minutes can help soothe tight muscles and prevent them from squeezing off circulation.

- Set a regular bedtime. Too much or too little sleep can trigger an aching head.

- Let Joe handle it. If you're taking aspirin to dull the pain, take it with coffee; the caffeine will speed absorption of the aspirin.

When to see a doctor: Any time a headache persists for more than 72 hours or prevents you from doing normal activities or is accompanied by vision problems, difficulty talking, coordination trouble, weakness in your arms and legs, difficulty thinking clearly, fever or vomiting.

Headaches accompanied by these symptoms can be a sign of high blood pressure, brain hemorrhage, stroke, brain tumor, meningitis or Lyme disease. Extremely intense pain that lasts as long as two hours once or twice a day, then abates suddenly could indicate cluster headaches. They can usually be alleviated with pure-oxygen therapy or headache-relieving prescription drugs.

9. Heartburn. The feeling of heartburn and the feeling of a heart attack are really not the same. Heartburn produces a fiery sensation when stomach acid seeps back up into the esophagus.

A heart attack is more a feeling of tightness in the chest as the heart muscle falters. Whatever you think you have, if it's accompanied by shortness of breath or sweating, assume it's serious.

When to see a doctor: Taking an antacid doesn't calm the fire within 15 minutes; heartburn is chronic or makes your stomach so sensitive that eating makes you feel ill. Any of these symptoms could be a sign of an ulcer or a type of hernia in which a small portion of the stomach slips through an opening in the diaphragm—the muscle that separates the chest and the abdomen and assists in breathing.

10. Lower-back pain. It feels serious, but back pain usually means simply that the muscles in your torso are tight or weak. In those cases, applying either ice or heat can alleviate the pain, but the most effective treatment is movement, in the form of exercises that shore up spine-supporting muscles in the abdomen and back, and stretches that keep lower-back muscles flexible.

When to see a doctor: Take a simple test—while lying on a firm mattress, straighten one leg and raise it 90 degrees. If pain shoots down your leg, seek medical help; you may have suffered a slip or injury of a disk, the jellylike cushion that works as a shock absorber between the vertebrae. Also see a doctor if pain lasts more than 72 hours or is so severe that it interferes with your work; you may require prescription painkillers or over-the-counter anti-inflammatories.

11. Nosebleed. You don't have to be a character from *Raging Bull* to suffer nosebleeds. The inside of the nose is lined with hundreds of tiny blood vessels that are vulnerable to trauma. So vulnerable, in fact, that a mere sneeze can start the blood flowing if, for example, the air is too cold and dry. Still, 5 to 10 percent of nosebleeds need a doctor's care, because of underlying problems like allergies and nasal infections. Nosebleeds can also be caused by taking certain medications, including aspirin, ibuprofen and some anti-arthritis drugs.

When to see a doctor: Nosebleeds are recurrent or produce gushes that won't stop even after you have pinched the nostrils closed for five minutes; the nosebleed starts with blood going down the back of your throat rather than out of your nose. A high-volume nosebleed may be a sign of high blood pressure, and repeated nosebleeds could indicate a clotting problem.

12. Red eyes. Irritation triggered by things like allergens or chlorinated pool water is a likely cause of redness, as is a broken blood vessel from straining under a heavy weight. As a general rule, if the eyes are irritated, don't rub them—that'll just aggravate the problem. Instead, try a cold compress or look for "eye decongestant" drops that constrict blood vessels (vasoconstrictors) and remove the red. (Some brands include an antihistamine that counteracts allergic itchiness and swelling.)

Using vasoconstrictors longer than four days could give you "rebound redness," because the blood vessels react to the drug by overdilating. If you wear contacts, keep infections at bay by cleaning and disinfecting your lenses every time you remove them, using fresh solutions. Use only the commercial contact lens preparations recommended for your hard or soft lenses and make sure to clean the cases, too.

When to see a doctor: If the redness persists for two or more days or is accompanied by thick or yellowish discharge, you may have a contagious condition called pinkeye, a bacterial infection that attacks the transparent membrane lining the eyelids and covering the eyeball. If you wear contact lenses, and redness persists for two or more hours after removing your contacts, you may have a bacterial or viral infection called keratitis. Contact lenses block oxygen from the eye, encouraging bacterial or viral growth. Both conditions can be treated with antibiotics.

13. Seeing spots. After age 50, it's common to see "floaters" along your field of vision—small dark drifting specks that are harmless bits of your eyeball's inner fluid. You're particularly prone to them if you're nearsighted, says Jason Slakter, M.D., eye specialist at the Manhattan Eye, Ear and Throat Hospital. More often than not, says Dr. Slakter, the spots eventually disappear on their own or your brain suppresses the image. You may not even notice them unless you're fatigued.

When to see a doctor: If floaters are persistent, seek medical attention. They could be telling you that you have an inflammation or infection within your eye or elsewhere in your body. This is especially true if the spots are accompanied by blurred or shadowy vision or start after you receive a blow to the head or eye. Frequent floaters could also mean a torn retina, a problem that, left untreated, could threaten your sight.

14. Stomach pain. Indigestion? Probably. Another possibility is an ulcer, either in your stomach (peptic) or in your intestines (duodenal). One sign of an ulcer that distinguishes it from less dire gastric distress is that an ulcer can actually be relieved for a short time by eating. Another cause of abdominal pain is *irritable bowel syndrome*, in which the intestines have trouble moving your food from its point of entry to its point of exit.

A telltale sign is recurrent abdominal pain accompanied by diarrhea or constipation and bloating. The pain will usually subside after a trip to the bathroom.

When to see a doctor: Stomach pain that is only temporarily relieved by eating could well be an ulcer and should be tended to. Pain that is sudden and severe, or lasts more than four days, may indicate gallbladder problems, appendicitis or other digestive diseases, or food poisoning.

15. Testicular pain. "Having acute scrotal pain requires you to see the doctor right away, because you could lose the testicle if it's not corrected in just a few hours," says Bruce H. Blank, M.D., a clinical associate professor of urology at Oregon Health Sciences University School of Medicine in Portland. In the case of torsion, a condition in which the testicle twists on the spermatic cord to which it's attached, the organ essentially strangles for lack of blood. (Try to stop squirming, please.) More common in adults is a bacterial infection of the epididymis, a spaghetti-like tube coiled up behind the testicle inside the scrotum.

The bacteria is sometimes transmitted by sexual intercourse, but any form of bacteria may cause it, including the kind that also causes urinary infections. When the epididymis is infected, a lump will emerge inside the scrotum, which may be red and feel hot to the touch.

When to see a doctor: See one immediately any time you suffer persistent testicular or scrotal pain, especially if it's accompanied by swelling, nausea, vomiting, abdominal pain, redness, abnormal discharge or difficulty urinating. Testicular cancer often develops as a lump, and any abnormality should be looked into.

—*Richard Allan*

Unusual Suspects

Many common health problems have unusual, even surprising causes. Here are some of the most likely causes that you'd never suspect.

•••••••••••••••••••••

PLENTY OF EVERYDAY HEALTH PROBLEMS don't take a medical degree to understand. Running a fever? Must have been that guy who sneezed all over you in the elevator. Stomachache? Maybe you should have passed on the third helping of takeout. Trace the cause and you can usually figure out the solution.

But there are also plenty of ailments that have less obvious causes, things you'd never suspect if somebody didn't warn you about them. We're talking about minor aches and pains and health glitches, problems that you really can cure or resolve without a doctor's help . . . if only you know what the problem is. To round up these unusual suspects, we interviewed doctors and combed through the medical literature as well as our own research files. Here's what we found.

BACKACHE

Your wallet. Sitting on your wallet can put pressure on your sciatic nerve, the major nerve running through the buttocks. The result, for many men, is lower-back pain.

Cowboy boots. They have a higher heel than other shoes, which can put *twice* as much stress on your back as you're used to, say researchers at Lehigh University in Bethlehem, Pennsylvania. Before you go doing the Achy Breaky, put cushioned inserts—available at any drugstore—in your boots. They can reduce impact to your joints and spine by up to 40 percent.

Smoking. Cigarettes and cigars reduce the amount of oxygen that travels to your spinal discs. This lack of oxygen can cause back pain. "If you smoke a pack of cigarettes a day, you'll probably double the amount of back pain you would have if you didn't smoke," says Brent Lovejoy, D.O., an occupational medicine specialist in Denver.

FATIGUE

Breathing. Guys who breathe through their mouths often are tired without knowing why. The reason is that mouth breathing tends to be shallow and rapid, and your body works too hard for the oxygen it gets, says Robert Fried, Ph.D., director of the Stress and Biofeedback Clinic of the Institute for Rational Emotive Therapy in New York City. You can remedy this problem by making a conscious effort to breathe slowly and steadily through your nose.

Not enough stress. While it's obvious that too much stress can take the wind out of your sails, experts also believe that you can get fatigued without *enough* stress. Paul J. Rosch, M.D., president of the American Institute of Stress in Yonkers, says a lack of stress leaves men feeling bored and not motivated. So if the job isn't enough to keep you hopping, add some stress by becoming a volunteer or tackling another chore that challenges you.

Shooting. Researchers in Colorado found that hunters and others who frequently use firearms have up to eight times more lead in their system—from lead dust in ammunition—and that can cause fatigue. This isn't a problem for the occasional hunter or marksman, but if you regularly go to shooting ranges, opt for copper- or nylon-jacketed ammo instead of the traditional pure-lead bullets.

• •

The Morning Disk Jockey

You may be able to ward off lower-back pain simply by waiting an hour after you wake up before starting vigorous exercise, such as running or weight lifting. When you're sleeping, fluid pools in your spinal disks, making your lower back tight, says Augustus A. White, M.D., a specialist in spine surgery at Beth Israel Hospital in Boston. That means you're most sensitive to irritation right after you get out of bed. Simply walking around for about an hour heads off backaches by squeezing that fluid out and making your back more limber. If you're in a hurry to start your workout, you can try performing some other light exercises to help speed up the drainage process: Sit in a chair, feet flat on the floor and gently bend forward, or stand with your hands on your hips and lean slightly from side to side.

BAD BREATH

Cooking. Even *handling* garlic can result in halitosis. That's because aromatic substances in the herb enter your body through pores in your hands, travel through your bloodstream and get released into your lungs before being exhaled, says Ronald S. Bogdasarian, M.D., of the University of Michigan in Ann Arbor. If you have to touch the stuff and halitosis sets in, try chewing parsley. It can keep breath fresh for up to 24 hours.

Your medications. Many prescription and over-the-counter drugs also cause bad breath by drying up saliva. Antihistamines, decongestants, diuretics, anti-anxiety drugs and even some heart medications lead the list.

If you take any of these, increase your intake of water or eat an orange to keep saliva flowing. Chewing gum or sucking on hard candies also helps.

BLOODSHOT EYES

Contact lens cleaner. Preservatives in contact lens cleaners can turn eyes redder than watching *Old Yeller*. So if you notice more eye redness than in the past, switch to a cleaner labeled "preservative-free."

"Red-out" products. Eyedrops that promise to remove redness can cause a rebound effect—meaning your eyes become red if you *don't* use them. This could occur if you use these products for more than four consecutive days, says Eric Donnenfeld, M.D., an associate professor of ophthalmology at North Shore University Hospital/Cornell Medical College in New York City.

Remove redness by placing a warm washcloth over your eyes if they don't itch, and a cool washcloth if they do itch. (Itching indicates an allergy, and coolness shrinks the blood vessels, says Dr. Donnenfeld.)

COLD SORES

Beer. The herpes simplex virus that causes these painful blisters on the lips and mouth needs the amino acid arginine to initiate its dirty work. Beer is rich in arginine, as are chocolate, cola, peas, peanuts and cashews. Limiting your intake of these foods may help reduce outbreaks if you are prone to them.

CHARLEY HORSE

Diet. If you get cramps in your calf or thigh at odd times—like while you're lying in bed—it could be the result of a magnesium deficiency, says Stephen Subotnick, D.P.M., a sports podiatrist in Hayward, California. Try eating foods rich in magnesium, such as halibut, mackerel, rice bran, tofu and spinach.

HEADACHE

Fluorescent lights. One common cause of headache is over your head—literally. That's because this popular choice of lighting actually flickers about 60 times a second. While this constant flickering is unnoticeable to the naked eye, it can cause headache and fatigue, according to research by Robert A. Baron, Ph.D., an industrial psychologist. If you work under fluorescent light (and who doesn't, since it's the most common lighting in offices), try to offset its effects with a table lamp or other incandescent lighting.

Sleeping on your stomach. "Headache can be caused by sleeping in an awkward position—even on your stomach—because the muscles in your neck contract," says Seymour Diamond, M.D., executive director of the National Headache Foundation and director of the Diamond Headache Clinic in Chicago. "Sleeping on your back is the best thing you can do, but many of my patients who are restless sleepers find relief with a Walpin pillow, which is hollowed in the middle to help your neck." You'll find this pillow at some drugstores and surgical supply stores.

VISION PROBLEMS

Tight collars. Shirt collars one-half inch too small can give you eyestrain, according to researchers at Cornell University in Ithaca, New York. The problem occurs because restricted blood flow to the head impairs the workings of the retina. Luckily, there's an easy solution: buy shirts that fit.

INSOMNIA

Nightcaps. Alcohol helps you *fall* asleep, but it doesn't keep you there. "Its sleep-inducing effects wear off very quickly," says Alex Clerk, M.D., director of the Sleep Disorders Clinic at Stanford University. "Often people who have taken a nightcap wake up in the middle of the night and then cannot get back to sleep. Even when it doesn't cause you to wake up, studies show alcohol fragments your sleep, so you don't wake up refreshed."

TENNIS ELBOW

Your racket. A racket with a metal frame can transmit the shock of ball contact to your elbow. Over time, that can strain your forearm tendons and make your elbow feel like it's been beaten by Pete Sampras in straight sets. Remedy: Get yourself a composition or graphite racket, which absorbs the shock better than metal.

Your swing. If you are leading with your elbow on your backhand, you are putting undue strain on your tendons, says Susan Perry, a physical therapist specializing in sports medicine at the Fort Lauderdale Sports Medicine Clinic in Florida. A properly executed backhand stroke gets your racket in front of your elbow.

IMPOTENCE

Underwear. This may come as quite a shock, but researchers in Cairo found that wearing polyester underwear can cause impotence—because of static electricity generated by manmade materials. Even cotton-poly blends can result in a "slight downturn in ability," according to the researchers, while 100-percent-cotton shorts have no effect.

Your diet. Just as a high-fat, high-cholesterol diet plays havoc with your heart, it can do similar damage to your penis. "Plaque from a bad diet and sedentary lifestyle can line the walls of the arteries in and to your penis, reducing blood flow and causing impotence," says Mark Cline, Ph.D., a researcher at the Male Health Center in Dallas. The good news is that adopting a healthy diet can reverse this situation, increasing blood flow and making for better erections.

STOMACHACHE

Your belt. A common cause of indigestion is wearing the belt too tight. Loosen it and you might find that the double pepperoni pizza wasn't entirely to blame. A doctor writing in the *Archives of Internal Medicine* says many middle-age men come to him complaining of mysterious heartburn and stomach cramps. In most cases, he says, it's caused by wearing belts or trousers too tightly.

Hot tea. Any beverage that's too hot or too cold can send your stomach into a spasm. Give your morning coffee a few moments to cool down before chugging it.

INFERTILITY

Your timing. Probably the biggest mistake couples trying to conceive make is to assume that a man's first ejaculation after abstaining from sex for a week or more is his best. "Usually, the *second* specimen is better, both in sperm count and motility," says Arthur L. Wisot, M.D., a fertility specialist in Redondo Beach, California. His advice: Make your first try two days before your partner starts ovulating and then go for the gold when she *is* ovulating.

Your position. Save the acrobatics for some other time. Studies show that the missionary position assures better contact of semen with the cervix, which can make a difference in marginal cases, says Dr. Wisot.

Hot water. A hot bath lowers sperm count and motility. So the would-be dad should stick with lukewarm showers and stay out of hot tubs.

—*Sid Kirchheimer*

The Prostate Controversy

Doctors are holding back treatment for prostate cancer—a matter of life and death for one in ten men. Some men are wondering why.

• • • • • • • • • • • • • • • • • • •

THE THING ABOUT THE PROSTATE IS, almost every man someday has to deal with it or, at minimum, think about dealing with it. Never mind that it's a small nodule of a thing no bigger than a walnut, tucked discreetly out of the way in the nether regions of the male anatomy. The prostate has a capacity for hitting us right where we live with troubles that are completely out of proportion to its diminutive size and quiet disposition. The prostate is so unassuming, in fact, that the worst malady it can produce, prostate cancer, can afflict you for years without provoking any symptoms whatsoever. But despite the silent nature of prostate cancer, the whole business of dealing with it is rapidly becoming a big, loud problem at the national level. Prostate care has become an issue for men—just as breast cancer is for women—and if you don't know what's at stake, we're here to tell you.

Cancer is at the crux of the matter, because it's the prostate problem that's likeliest to kill you. And it kills men in a big way. In 1993 the disease killed 35,000 American men. It's the second leading cancer killer of men, behind lung cancer. But while male deaths from lung cancer have started to decline, the death rate from prostate cancer is climbing, with a 17 percent increase since the 1960s. One reason is that men are living longer. In fact, experts say that if you live long enough, you are almost sure to develop prostate cancer.

In recent years, a number of important advances have been made in detecting and treating prostate cancer. The most talked about discovery is a simple but sensitive blood check called the prostate-specific antigen (PSA) test, which makes it easier for doctors to accurately diagnose the disease in its earliest stages. When prostate cancer is caught early, the cure rate is 91 percent. It's no wonder the PSA test has strong advocates in the health profession and is considered a major improvement over previous methods of screening.

UNBELIEVABLE BUT TRUE

Yet, incredible as it may sound, many doctors feel men shouldn't take advantage of the PSA blood check. "The struggle between these two schools will be a male health battleground throughout the entire decade of the 1990s," says William Catalona, M.D., chief of the urologic surgery division at Washington University's Barnes Hospital in St. Louis.

The critics say that the PSA test is basically too sensitive, that it detects cancers not yet advanced enough to warrant concern. If the idea of cancer not warranting concern sounds odd, consider the example of a 50-year-old man whose PSA readings indicate a very early stage tumor. Had the PSA test not come along, he might not have had his cancer detected for another 15 years. In fact, though one in ten are destined to get the disease, 80 percent of cases are not diagnosed until age 65 or older. Now that our 50-year-old knows it's there, he may choose to have surgery to remove it. Would he be acting too soon? This is a pertinent question for two reasons. First, prostate surgery carries with it the chance of some devastating side effects—impotence or incontinence or both. Second, studies suggest that up to 75 percent of patients with prostate cancer die of other causes before their prostate cancer ever becomes a significant threat.

These are the key points in the PSA debate: Those who favor testing say men have a right to early diagnosis and prompt treatment, and the don't-test doctors argue that there's no point in risking years of potential misery to eliminate a cancer that may never ail you.

UNDERSTANDING THE PROSTATE

To understand the questions surrounding testing, it helps to know what the prostate gland does and what else can go wrong with it. If the penis is a cannon, the prostate is the ammunition loader. Its function is to produce seminal fluid and release it during ejaculation. If you put your finger on your abdomen just above the point at which the penis protrudes from the body, you'll get a good idea of where the prostate sits deep inside, just below the bladder and in front of the rectum.

It's also important to understand that the two most common prostate problems usually aren't life threatening, although they can be exceedingly high on the annoyance scale. These are *prostatitis*, an inflammation of the prostate gland often caused by infection, and *benign prostatic hyperplasia* (BPH), a condition in which the prostate goes through a growth spurt, usually after age 40. The newly enlarged prostate presses against the urethra, making urination difficult. By some estimates, more than half of men over age 60 have enlarged prostates, and 80 percent of 80-year-olds do. Though its very name includes the word benign, you may have heard that BPH is a risk factor for prostate cancer. In fact, the consensus now is that the two have nothing to do with one another.

What BPH and prostate cancer do have in common is that they generally occur in older men. Which brings us back to our debate. The argument that prostate cancer isn't worth troubling about because it usually hits so late in life can be deceptive for active men. "Men are living longer and staying in better shape than they used to," Dr. Catalona says, pointing out that the longer you live, the more likely it is that prostate cancer will catch up with you. "My feeling is that there's a general attitude that prostate cancer is an old man's disease, so we shouldn't get too excited about it," he says. "But to suggest that this is not an important problem is ridiculous."

For years, the standard recommendation has been that men get screened annually for prostate cancer starting at age 50, or age 40 for higher-risk men such as African Americans and those with a family history of the disease. (See "Where Do You

• •

Through Abstinence Comes Accuracy

Sometimes, painful sacrifices must be made in the interest of health. For example, abstaining from sex for a week before a prostate cancer blood screening may give you more accurate test results. Researchers at New York City's Memorial Sloan-Kettering Cancer Center found that levels of prostate-specific antigen, the key marker of the cancer, were misleadingly low in men who ejaculated before the test.

Stand in the Risk Pool?" on page 169.) Getting screened centered on having your doctor conduct a digital-rectal exam (DRE). Digital means finger (the doctor's, gloved), and rectal... well, you get the picture. It's not the most pleasant procedure in the world, and many men shunned it.

Then, Dr. Catalona did a pioneering study demonstrating the effectiveness of PSA testing. PSA is a protein in seminal fluid. It is made only in the prostate, but circulates throughout the body, so a blood sample can give you an idea of how much of it the gland is cranking out at any given time. Because more PSA gets into the bloodstream when problems arise, elevated levels are an early warning signal for cancer. In one study, Dr. Catalona found that PSA screening detects almost twice the number of potentially curable cancers as does the DRE.

STANDARD CARE CONTROVERSY

The American Cancer Society now recommends that annual screenings include both the DRE and a PSA test, which costs about $50. "That's really become the standard of care," says Richard E. Greenberg, M.D., chief of urologic oncology at Fox Chase Cancer Center in Philadelphia.

The National Cancer Institute (NCI), the federal government's cancer-research agency, currently only recommends the DRE. The reason is that it wants more evidence that catching this slow-growing cancer sooner makes a difference. "Early detection doesn't necessarily mean you'll live any longer," says John Gohagan, Ph.D., chief of NCI's early-detection branch.

The proof positive some researchers are looking for won't be available until the completion of a 16-year-long national cancer screening study. "Half a million men are going to die of prostate cancer while they're waiting for the results of this study," says Dr. Catalona. "I feel that a lot of those who are against PSA screening are experts from other fields who don't see real patients and are dealing with this issue in an abstract sense."

But it needs to be said at this point that no one claims the PSA test is perfect. About 9 percent of men who get an all-clear reading actually do have prostate cancer. And because PSA also rises in response to lesser problems such as BPH, up to three-quarters of men who get an elevated reading don't have cancer.

"That's why you want both the PSA and the DRE," says urologist Joseph E. Oesterling, M.D., an associate professor at the Mayo Clinic in Rochester, Minnesota, and editor-in-chief of the journal *Urology*. "The PSA can pick up cancers that the DRE can't and vice versa." Dr. Oesterling and others note, though, that if you had to choose between one or the other, the PSA test is clearly superior.

KNOWLEDGE IS POWER

So if your PSA test finds evidence of malignancy, what should you do? The first step is to try to relax. Prostate cancer generally moves very slowly, which means there's time to consider your options carefully and make informed decisions.

Part of being informed means knowing up front that the costs of not treating prostate cancer until its later stages can be quite high. Even men in the earliest stages of malignancy stand a 12 percent chance of dying from it if it goes untreated for ten years. And once the cancer has spread beyond the gland, the options remaining to you are extremely unappealing.

The most common late-stage treatments are designed to restrain the disease by robbing the body of testosterone, the male hormone that fuels the cancer's growth. The first choice is decidedly ugliest. It entails removing the testicles (castration), which make most of the male hormones. The second is monthly injections of other hormones or chemicals that block testosterone. Removing the testicles is most effective and least expensive. In either case, the lack of testosterone damps your sex drive and makes it less likely you'd be able to perform if you were interested.

There are plenty of options available before you ever get to that point, however, if you catch the cancer before it spreads.

Your initial course of action is determined by how high your PSA reading is. Interpretation of these readings has been substantially refined with research from the Mayo Clinic showing that it's natural for PSA levels to increase with age. This advance alone makes it less likely that older men will be subjected to costly and invasive diagnostic tests, and more likely that younger men will have dangerous cancers detected at an early and curable stage, according to Dr. Oesterling, who conducted the research. Where once the "normal" cutoff was 4 nanograms (billionths of a gram) per milliliter for all men, it's now 2.5 if you're in your forties, 3.5 in your fifties, 4.5 in your sixties and 6.5 in your seventies.

FIND OUT MORE

For men whose readings are high, the immediate goal is to find out more about the cancer, starting with confirmation that it exists. If the digital-rectal exam discovers nothing, a transrectal ultrasound test may be done to detect small tumors that your doctor can't feel. If you still come up clean, most doctors recommend putting off further action until you get another PSA in several months. There's a chance your PSA will stay the same or even be lower the next time around.

If cancer is suspected, the next step is a needle biopsy, a procedure your urologist can do in his office. The biopsy extracts tiny samples of the prostate to be examined under a microscope, which gives the doctor an inkling of how aggressive your tumor is. If it's a fairly tame tumor, here, too, you may want to put off any action while monitoring your condition to see if it gets worse, an option known as watchful waiting. You may want to continue monitoring your PSA for years before taking any more drastic steps, especially if your levels remain constant.

If the tumor is aggressive, however, particularly if you're healthy and young (say, under 60), you'll want to consider a prostatectomy to remove the cancerous gland. Another option is radiation, which is almost as effective but which also carries the risks of causing impotence and incontinence.

Before making a final decision, though, you should weigh critical factors such as your age, your health, your family medical history or anything else having to do with your life expectancy. As a rule, you need at least ten good years left in you to make the risks of the operation worth taking. "I'm reluctant to operate on any man over age 70," says Kenneth Goldberg, M.D., founder and director of the Male Health Center in Dallas.

If you and your doctor feel you'd benefit from surgery, you'll be glad to know that your chances of retaining potency have substantially improved over the past decade, thanks to a technique that spares the nerves needed for an erection and an orgasm. Before this new operation came along, the surgery rendered all men impotent. Now, the method's inventor,

Patrick Walsh, M.D., director of the Brady Urological Institute at Johns Hopkins University in Baltimore, says that 90 percent of his patients younger than age 50 can still have erections sufficient for intercourse after recovering fully from the surgery (a process that may take one to two years). For men in their fifties, the figure drops to 75 percent, and for men in their sixties, 60 percent. Keep in mind, however, that Dr. Walsh is reputed to be the best prostate surgeon in the country; other doctors say your chances of remaining potent under age 65 are closer to 50/50. So when considering surgery, be sure to take into account the potential for lifestyle-altering side effects.

Hopefully, getting a prostatectomy will provide the last word on your cancer. When doctors open you up, they sample the nearby lymph nodes to see if the cancer has metastasized (spread) beyond the prostate. (This sampling can also be done in a separate operation, using special tools and cameras inserted through small holes in the abdomen.) If they find any signs that it has spread, most doctors will leave your prostate in; there's little point in taking it out because doing so will no longer cure the cancer. At that juncture, unfortunately, nothing will.

With the potential costs of waiting too long while an invisible cancer advances, it's easy to see why so many urologists so strongly advocate early detection. "There are many men I believe I've saved because their cancer was caught early," Dr. Goldberg says. "And whatever your doctor recommends, it never hurts to get a second opinion."

A GODSEND

"The PSA test has been a godsend to me," says Richard J. Howe, Ph.D., retired president of Pennzoil and a spokesman for the men's advocacy group Us Too. "Without it, I probably would not have been diagnosed for years. And I, for one, was willing to deal with the side effects of surgery in exchange for a possible cure."

It's always better to know than not to know, says Dr. Goldberg. "The bottom line is, if your life expectancy is good, take care of yourself—eat right, exercise regularly and get regular checkups, including the PSA. One reason men don't live longer than women is because they don't go for exams more often."

WHERE DO YOU STAND IN THE RISK POOL?

A number of factors have been linked to higher rates of prostate cancer. Here's the lowdown on a few of the most important.

Vasectomy. The National Institutes of Health have concluded that the weak links found to date are likely due to chance or "detection bias," meaning men with vasectomies may simply see their urologists more.

Race. Black men get prostate cancer at a 40 percent higher rate than whites do. Researchers speculate it may have to do with blacks' synthesizing less vitamin D, low levels of which have also been associated with the disease.

Family history. Having a father or a brother with the disease doubles your risk; having two members of your immediate family stricken at an early age (mid-fifties or younger) raises your risk to five times the average.

High-fat diet. Several studies have established a link between fat intake and prostate cancer. Research from Harvard University suggests that diets high in animal fats can significantly raise your risk for developing *advanced* prostate cancer. In a study of over 47,000 men, those who ate high-fat diets were 1.8 times more likely to have a case of prostate cancer that had spread or was diagnosed as fatal than their low-fat-eating counterparts. And when the primary source of that fat was red meat (beef, lamb, pork), their risk for developing advanced cancer more than doubled. Other high-fat foods implicated were bacon, butter, mayonnaise and creamy salad dressings.

Researchers suggest that a high-fat diet may act as a type of environmental trigger for the disease. While family history and race could make you more likely to *develop* prostate cancer, eating less red meat and other fatty foods may ultimately give you a better chance of surviving it. Other dietary choices that may help lower your risk include soy products and high-fiber foods, such as beans, lentils, tomatoes, peas and dried fruit.

Lack of exercise. Preliminary studies suggest regular vigorous activities like brisk walking and sports lower your risk, perhaps by lowering the body's testosterone levels.

—Richard Laliberte

Blood and Numbers

Have we been looking at the wrong cholesterol numbers all along? Here are the latest facts.

• • • • • • • • • • • • • • • • • • •

A SCORE OF OVER 200 may be desirable if you're a bowler, but it may not seem so hot if it's the number that comes up on your cholesterol test. Research, however, indicates the old way of measuring cholesterol may be misleading. In fact, a rising tide of evidence shows that one particular component of your cholesterol makeup can be as important as the total number in the fight against heart disease.

That's pretty good news for the nearly half of us in the United States with cholesterol levels above the 200 mark. It may also be a warning to those of us who thought we had heart disease licked because we've kept our total cholesterol scores low. Fortunately, there are steps we can all take to improve our cholesterol profile and hold our risk of heart disease to a minimum.

What's highly important, experts say, is your level of high-density lipoprotein (HDL), the "good" cholesterol component. The government's National Cholesterol Education Program has issued new recommendations that doctors should measure HDL whenever they test for cholesterol and should consider the measurement in planning treatment for their patients.

DON'T BE MISLED

Its clear from evidence that measuring total cholesterol alone can be misleading. "Up to 40 percent of heart attack victims have been reported to have a total cholesterol under 200," says Peter Wood, Ph.D., professor of medicine at Stanford University School of Medicine. A significant proportion of these patients also have low HDL levels, and he says that's the missing link. So important are HDLs to heart health that when levels get high enough—above the 60 mark—they become a huge plus, neutralizing such negative risks as diabetes or high blood pressure, says William Hazzard, M.D., chairman of the department of medicine at the Bowman Gray School of Medicine in Winston-Salem, North Carolina.

Here's how it works. Cholesterol is a white, waxy substance found in meat, eggs and dairy foods. You wouldn't want to eliminate the stuff entirely; your body requires it to sheathe cells. But excess cholesterol also collects in the bloodstream, where, like former Soviet satellite countries, it breaks into rival factions and gets involved in a dirty little war. The low-density lipoproteins (LDL) are the bad guys, the vessel-cloggers, that lay siege to your health by depositing fat-laden bunkers on the walls of your arteries. The HDLs are the repelling forces tasked with patrolling the vessels and rousting the evil LDLs.

THE KEY RATIO

While it's useful to know your total cholesterol count and your individual HDL and LDL levels, the key to identifying your risk for heart disease is your total-to-HDL ratio. To find it, divide your total cholesterol by your HDL measurement. Keep this number at 4.5 or less and you're in good shape. For example, even if total cholesterol is 240, you're not at risk if your HDL is 54 or above.

If the ratio *is* above 4.5, ask your doctor to help you pinpoint the problem. You can then plan your attack on two fronts: lowering your total cholesterol while trying to preserve and even raise HDL levels. We're not talking about splitting atoms here. "Give yourself four to eight weeks and you can easily drop your total cholesterol 8 to 15 percent (20 to 30 points), without drugs, often while raising the beneficial HDL," says Basil Rifkind, M.D., chief of the Lipid Metabolism and Atherogenesis Branch of the National Heart, Lung and Blood Institute in Bethesda, Maryland.

It's likely that you already know the principal steps for lowering total cholesterol. Here's a refresher course.

- Reduce intake of cholesterol-rich foods like red meat and dairy products. Also limit yourself to three whole eggs per week, including those in baked and other prepared foods.

- Replace saturated fats like butter with vegetable spreads and monounsaturated fats such as olive oil.

- Eat more fruits and vegetables. In one study, 310 people who had heart disease and ate fruits and vegetables before major meals raised HDL levels by nearly 6 percent.

- Focus on water-soluble fiber. That special fiber scours the arteries of loitering LDLs and ushers them from the body. Excellent sources are beans; grains like oats, barley, corn and rice brans; and fruits containing pectin, like apples and strawberries.

The blueprint for raising HDL is different. "While LDL cholesterol responds primarily to diet, HDL levels are most responsive to weight loss and exercise," says Thomas Kottke, M.D., professor of medicine in the Mayo Clinic's Division of Cardiovascular Diseases in Rochester, Minnesota. Below are the best, and least painful, ways to boost HDL cholesterol—while still forcing those annoying LDLs into exile.

Get moving. Aerobic exercise will bolster HDL, but if you're not one for an early-morning jog, consider this: Just walking 30 to 45 minutes three times a week will do the job. Add clubs, balls and ugly pants and you've got golf; in one study, men with normal to mildly elevated cholesterol levels who played golf three times a week significantly improved their cholesterol profiles.

Pump a little iron. And we do mean a little. While those palookas straining under 295 pounds of metal aren't helping their cholesterol levels, moderate-weight, high-repetition strength training can pump up your HDL score by as much as 11 percent, according to a study at Florida State University in Tallahassee.

Steer away from smoke. Smoking has long been known to depress HDL levels. Researchers have found that just hanging around human chimneys can do the same thing. In a study of 391 students, nonsmokers exposed to high levels of secondhand smoke suffered almost a 7 percent drop in HDL levels compared with nonsmokers who were exposed to low levels.

Vent yourself. Studies by researchers at Brown University in Providence, Rhode Island, determined that men who scored the highest on repression in psychological tests measuring anxiety and defensiveness also had the highest cholesterol levels and the lowest HDL levels. This doesn't mean you should shout and scream, but it's clearly a mistake to suppress every emotion as men are wont to do, says Raymond Niaura, Ph.D., associate professor of psychiatry at Brown University School of Medicine in Providence, Rhode Island, and principal researcher of the study.

Drink a little. Although alcohol elicits groans from most doctors because of its potential for abuse, few experts can deny its HDL-boosting benefits. "Moderate consumption, by which I mean no more than one or two drinks a day, often improves your cholesterol profile," says Dr. Wood.

Go fish. It's common knowledge that diets high in mackerel, tuna, salmon and sardines help keep heart arteries clear by lowering levels of triglycerides (another component of your cholesterol profile with artery-clogging potential). Research is showing that getting hooked on fish—to the tune of seven ounces a day—can raise HDL by as much as 12 percent.

Get your share of vitamins and minerals. A study at Tufts University in Medford, Massachusetts, showed that people who consume 180 milligrams or more of vitamin C a day have 5 to 10 percent higher levels of HDL cholesterol than those with low amounts of vitamin C in their diets. Vitamin C is common in oranges, strawberries, grapefruit and broccoli. Other studies have shown that vitamin E (found in nuts, wheat germ and canola oil) and beta-carotene (found in carrots and spinach) may help prevent the buildup of artery-clogging plaque, while chromium (common in dried prunes and wheat germ) may also help lower cholesterol.

• •

Running Wide Open

Athletes have lower risk of heart disease, and one study sheds some light on why that may be. In a comparison of the coronary arteries of 22 men—11 marathon runners and 11 sofa spuds—the runners' arteries were capable of opening twice as wide as the nonexercisers'. One possible explanation: Arteries that open wider can provide more blood to the heart and are less likely to clog shut.

Try natural medicine. Some men who aren't responsive to diet and exercise will be put on a drug regimen by their doctors. Should drugs be in your future, first ask your doctor about niacin, an inexpensive B vitamin that can yield druglike results when taken in high doses. In a study of 34 men with heart disease and low levels of HDL, daily 2,400-milligram doses of niacin raised HDL levels 30 percent in three months. (Do not attempt this therapy unless under a doctor's supervision because of the occasionally dangerous side effects.)

—*David Zinczenko*

Your Home Pharmacy

You no longer need a prescription for some of the most effective pain relievers and other medicines. Here's a handy home guide.

• • • • • • • • • • • • • • • • • •

YOU'RE SICK WITH A BAD HEAD COLD. The kind that makes you contemplate the guillotine. But that would take too much effort. Besides, you're a do-it-yourself kind of guy. So you trudge off to the local 24-hour drug warehouse for relief. And there you're confronted with aisles and rows and stacks of medications for every conceivable ailment from "Arrgrumph" to "Zoacanthosis." In the middle, you spy the cold remedies: syrups, elixirs, capsules and tabs, in "regular," "extra" and "maximum" strengths, plus those multisymptom remedies that claim to cure everything but baldness. Which should you grab? Choosing wisely may seem like a daunting task. There are more than 125,000 nonprescription drug products on the market. On one visit to a drugstore, we counted 47 cold and flu remedies, 27 allergy medicines and 35 pain relievers. Fortunately, that cornucopia of cures is made up mostly of different brands, strengths or combinations of a few core drugs. If you know what's ailing you and what active ingredients will fix the problem, you can make an informed choice.

Of course, you shouldn't attempt a drugstore fix for every illness. As a general rule, for severe symptoms or a problem that lasts more than a few days, see a physician. Another thing: always read the label. Men, in particular, tend to have problems with medications, because they don't like to follow directions, says Roger Maickel, Ph.D., professor of pharmacology and toxicology at Purdue University in West Lafayette, Indiana. "They adhere to the American philosophy that if two pills work well, four really ought to do the job. And they mix over-the-counter (OTC) drugs with prescription medications," which can have serious consequences.

But if you exercise a reasonable amount of caution, OTC remedies provide quick and inexpensive relief for many common health problems. Below is a guide to help you negotiate the myriad of nonprescription medicines at your local drug emporium.

ACHES AND PAINS

There are a lot of pain relievers out there. But whether you're hurting from a headache or too much touch football, drugstore relief comes in one of three drugs: aspirin, acetaminophen and ibuprofen. Picking the right one for you is easy once you know what each does best.

Aspirin has been relieving pain ever since American Indians chewed willow bark to get at it in its raw form, salicylic acid. It works by blocking the body's output of chemicals that send pain messages to the brain.

Two standard 325-milligram tablets will ease mild to moderate headache pain, muscle aches and fevers. Pain relief aside, research has uncovered other properties of aspirin that are nothing short of amazing. Experts say that chewing and swallowing an aspirin tablet may actually reduce the impact of a heart attack in progress by preventing a blood clot from forming completely. And studies show that small daily doses (a quarter to half a tablet) can cut risk of heart attack and stroke by 30 and 25 percent respectively. There's also evidence that taking aspirin daily may help slash your chances of developing stomach and colon cancers. (Consult your doctor before starting any regular aspirin therapy.)

Aspirin's main drawback is that it causes stomach upset in up to 10 percent of users. One answer to this problem is to take your aspirin with milk or food. Another is to use coated aspirin, such as Ecotrin. The coating keeps the pill intact in your stomach; the aspirin doesn't dissolve until it reaches the small intestine. You get the same amount of drug in the bloodstream, but it can take two to three hours to get there. For that reason, coated aspirins are not the best cures for a pounding headache, says John Baum, M.D., professor of medicine and pediatrics at the University of Rochester School of Medicine and Dentistry in New York.

In that case, you might want acetaminophen, a pain reliever that's easy on the stomach. You'll recognize it by some common brand names—Tylenol and Aspirin-Free Anacin. Milligram for milligram, it does as good a job as aspirin of reducing fever and relieving aches, but because it lacks aspirin's anti-inflammatory power, it isn't as effective against sprained ankles or arthritis, where swelling adds to the throbbing pain.

If major joint aches and inflammation are your problem, you may want to reach for ibuprofen, a former prescription drug now sold generically or under brand names like Advil, Nuprin and Motrin IB. It's more expensive than aspirin and acetaminophen, but it's stronger. You get 200 milligrams in a one-pill regular dose.

Studies show that ibuprofen is the best pain reliever for many overexertion injuries such as tendinitis. In fact, a dose of ibuprofen taken prior to exercise has been found to lessen aches in little-used muscles. In one study, weekend warriors who had taken ibuprofen before exercising experienced 60 percent less muscle soreness compared with untreated sub-

• •

Kidney Punch

If you're prone to kidney stones, drink plenty of orange juice. Tests performed on men with kidney stones at the University of Texas Southwestern Medical Center in Dallas determined that drinking a little more than a quart of orange juice a day was nearly as effective at keeping kidney stones from forming as standard medication. The citrate in the juice inhibits formation of calcium stones, scientists say.

jects 24 hours after exercise. Experts caution, though, that pain is a natural warning signal. "Often soreness means you've done enough. It is not wise to block pain in advance," says Dr. Baum.

DIARRHEA

You cruise through a Cozumel vacation without a hitch— until the day of your return, when Montezuma exacts his famed revenge. Diarrhea is your body's natural attempt to get rid of unwanted bacteria. Experts caution against trying to curtail traveler's diarrhea before it has run its course, since the longer the bug stays in your stomach, the longer you'll be sick. But you have to take action sometimes—like when you are sandwiched between two large gentlemen on a seven-hour plane ride home.

The most effective antidiarrhea medicine you can buy is loperamide hydrochloride (Imodium A-D), a new OTC remedy that used to be a prescription drug. This powerful medicine shuts down nerve endings in the intestinal muscles so the intestines aren't triggered to expel their contents as quickly.

COLDS AND FLU

When a cold or flu strikes, all you can do is try to make yourself more comfortable by relieving the typical symptoms: sore throat, body aches, headache, sneezing, runny nose, fever and coughing. These symptoms may appear at different times as the virus runs its course, or they may bombard you all at once.

What you have to decide is whether you want to fight back with a rifle or a shotgun. The rifle approach targets a single symptom. For a sore throat, for example, you take an anesthetic lozenge. The shotgun approach attacks a field of symptoms by combining, say, a decongestant, an antihistamine, a cough suppressant and a pain reliever in a single preparation, as in Contac Severe Cold and Flu Formula, NyQuil LiquiCaps, Comtrex and many others.

The predominant view in health care is that the shotgun approach is wasteful. "A multisymptom remedy implies that you have those exact symptoms," says Thomas A. Gossel, Ph.D., professor of pharmacology and toxicology at Ohio Northern

University College of Pharmacy in Ada. Often you don't, so you end up getting unneeded medication. And paying for it.

Here's what to look for in cold remedies at your drugstore.

Throat soothers. If the soreness is deep in your throat, a squirt of an anesthetic spray like Chloraseptic may provide the quickest relief. Chloraseptic contains phenol, which kills the germs that are causing the pain and acts as a painkiller.

Lozenges. These offer longer-lasting relief because they dissolve slowly in your mouth, bathing your throat with pain-numbing medication each time you swallow. Best ingredients include benzocaine (Cepacol Anesthetic Lozenges), hexylresorcinol (Sucrets Cold Formula) and dyclonine hydrochloride (Sucrets Maximum Strength). Note: If you still have a sore throat after two to three days of sucking on lozenges, stop using them and visit a doctor.

Cough medicines. First, realize that coughing is good for you. It's your body's natural way of keeping your airways clear. If coughing is bringing up phlegm, you should keep it going—no matter how much your wife complains. You can help the process by taking an expectorant. The choice here is easy because the Food and Drug Administration (FDA) has recognized only one kind: guaifenesin, the stuff in scores of cold medicines. It works by stimulating glands to secrete more fluid, which in turn thins the mucus in your chest so it will be easier to cough up. "But guaifenesin is only as effective as the amount of water you take with it," says Dr. Gossel. "Drink as much as you can hold—a minimum of eight to ten glasses a day."

Don't expect an expectorant to stop a cough. It won't. If you have a dry, unproductive hack, you'll want a cough suppressant. Choose a lozenge, syrup or pill containing dextromethorphan (Hold DM cough suppressant lozenge, Vicks Formula 44), diphenhydramine hydrochloride (Benylin Cough Syrup) or codeine (available over the counter only in certain states). All these work by turning off the brain's cough center. Many experts agree that dextromethorphan is the safest and most effective.

Decongestants. That stuffy feeling in your nose comes from a swelling of your mucous membranes, usually triggered by a cold virus or an allergy. There are two good reasons for choosing spray decongestants over oral ones. First, they work faster, because they send the medicine directly where it's needed. Second, they have fewer side effects, since little of the drug is absorbed into the bloodstream.

When hunting for a decongestant spray, look for the ingredients oxymetazoline hydrochloride (Afrin, Dristan) or phenylephrine hydrochloride (Neo-Synephrine). These ease congestion by constricting swollen blood vessels in your nasal passages. You can use sprays for only three to five days. After that you run the risk of developing rebound congestion, a body reaction to stopping use of the sprays that can be worse than what you started with.

The oral decongestants, pseudoephedrine hydrochloride (Sudafed) and phenylpropanolamine hydrochloride (Allerest 12 Hour Caplets), can be used for a longer period of time. But be wary. They're stimulants and can produce such side effects as dry mouth, jitteriness, insomnia, high blood pressure and increased heart rate.

Antihistamines. The main weapons against hives and allergies, antihistamines also dry up nasal passages, effectively decreasing the sneezing, itching and runny nose associated with colds.

Some of the best-selling nonprescription antihistamines include brompheniramine maleate (Dimetane), chlorpheniramine maleate (Chlor-Trimeton), diphenhydramine hydrochloride (Benadryl, Benylin) and clemastine fumarate (Tavist 1).

All work quickly, but they tend to zonk you out. "To get around the sedative effect, try taking smaller doses during the day and save the full, therapeutic level for bedtime," says James Kemp, M.D., of the Allergy and Asthma Medical Group in San Diego.

Some cold and allergy remedies combine a decongestant and an antihistamine (Tavist D, Sudafed Plus, Dimetapp Extentabs), a tactic that makes sense since antihistamines alone won't clear up a stuffy nose. And the stimulating effect of the decongestant may somewhat offset the sleep-inducing effect of the antihistamine.

WARTS

These little cauliflower-shaped growths are caused by viruses, and they are highly contagious. If you get them, bring out the wart paint. The effective ingredient in OTC wart remedies is skin-peeling salicylic acid. It comes in 12 to 40 percent solutions, creams and patches. Compound-W, probably the most common product, contains 17 percent acid. For stubborn plantar warts, many dermatologists recommend a salicylic acid plaster, such as Mediplast, or the Trans-Ver-Sal transdermal patch, which delivers continuous doses of the drug for several hours. Check with your doctor before using these preparations as they can cause reactions in some people.

HEARTBURN/STOMACHACHE

For occasional heartburn, queasy stomach or stomachache from eating too much, an antacid can soothe your digestive distress. Most use one or a combination of the following ingredients to neutralize excess stomach acid: sodium bicarbonate (Alka-Seltzer), calcium carbonate (Tums), magnesium hydroxide (Phillips' Milk of Magnesia) or aluminum hydroxide (Mylanta).

A good rule of thumb is to stay away from those that are high in sodium (300 milligrams or more per dose), because salt can promote high blood pressure and water retention in sensitive individuals. Also, some people may find that calcium carbonate and aluminum compounds cause constipation. Others may notice that magnesium antacids cause diarrhea. As logic might suggest, if you tend to have trouble with constipation, pick a brand that lists magnesium first on the label. Or, if you're more prone to diarrhea, pick a brand listing calcium first, advises William B. Ruderman, M.D., chairman of the department of gastroenterology at the Cleveland Clinic-Florida in Fort Lauderdale.

Antacids are safe to take occasionally. Feeling the need to pop one after every meal, however, could signal a more serious problem, such as ulcers, that a physician should check out.

If you have gas with your upset stomach, try an antacid that includes the harmless antiflatulent chemical simethicone. Mylanta and Di-Gel are two examples. You can also buy antigas medication alone, such as Mylicon Gas or Gas-X.

MOTION SICKNESS

Nothing can ruin a cruise or a fishing trip quicker than a case of motion sickness. A number of drugs prevent the problem, and one of the most effective is Bonine, a chewable tablet that contains the antihistamine meclizine hydrochloride. A single 25- to 50-milligram dose is effective for up to 24 hours. Another good deterrent is dimenhydrinate (Dramamine). Just make sure you take it an hour or two before getting on the boat/plane/roller coaster. If you wait until you're queasy, you're too late.

ATHLETE'S FOOT/JOCK ITCH

Fungal infections on the skin start in warm, moist places, which is to say usually between your toes or between your legs. The fungus is the same in both places, and the two best drugs for attacking it are clotrimazole (Lotrimin AF) and miconazole nitrate (Micatin), says Stephen M. Schleicher, M.D.,

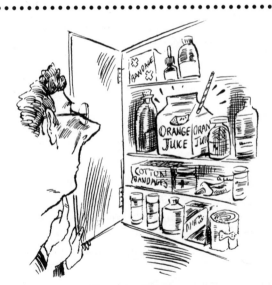

Orange Heals

Vitamin C speeds the healing of stubborn wounds, say researchers at Jefferson Medical College in Philadelphia. They applied a water solution containing 10 percent ascorbic acid to persistent bedsores of five patients. After a week of vitamin C treatment, the sores showed a significant increase in the amount of healed tissue.

MIXED TROUBLES

Combining certain drugs can create a dangerous cocktail.

While taking	Avoid	Reason
Anti-coagulants	Aspirin and ibuprofen	Mixture exaggerates blood-thinning effect and may cause bleeding. (heparin, warfarin)
Oral diabetes drugs	Aspirin	May boost drug's blood glucose-lowering effect.
Aspirin or ibuprofen	Alcoholic beverages	May damage stomach lining and cause bleeding.
Acetaminophen	Alcoholic beverages	May cause liver damage, especially in alcoholics.
Antihistamines	Alcoholic beverages	Antihistamines are sedatives; alcohol may increase drowsiness. Also, since both antihistamines and alcohol have a dehydrating effect on some glands, those with asthma, glaucoma or prostate problems should be particularly wary of this combination.

co-director of the Dermatology Center in Philadelphia. For a one-two punch, he recommends a daily treatment that includes sprinkling on a powder to aid drying, then applying an antifungal cream. Treated this way, mild jock itch normally clears up within two weeks and athlete's foot in three to four weeks.

HIVES/RASHES/POISON IVY

You're probably thinking of calamine lotion, that pink goo your mom smeared all over you when you were a kid. Sorry to say, the FDA has ruled it ineffective for itch relief.

You're better off using hydrocortisone creams such as Cortaid Maximum Strength. Hydrocortisone is a powerful anti-inflammatory agent that relieves swelling and consequently

While taking	Avoid	Reason
Oral decongestants	Caffeinated coffee and colas	Can produce nervousness, insomnia, rapid heartbeat.
Tetracycline or some high blood pressure medications	Antacids	Can keep some prescription drugs from being absorbed into the bloodstream, which renders them ineffective.
Many prescription drugs	Antidiarrheal products	Antidiarrheals can sweep other drugs that contain bulking agents through the digestive system before they reach the bloodstream.

itching. Another good remedy is a topical antihistamine such as diphenhydramine hydrochloride (Benadryl Anti-Itch). It works by blocking histamine from attaching to receptor cells in your skin and causing itching and rashes.

CONSTIPATION

You can get addicted to irritant laxatives containing phenolphthalein (Ex-Lax, Feen-A-Mint) to the point where you can't have a normal bowel movement without them, says Dr. Maickel. The chemical in these laxatives stimulates the nerves in the intestines to start their wavelike contractions. It's safer to remedy constipation with a natural bulk-forming laxative. You can do that by eating a high-fiber diet or taking a commercial laxative containing psyllium (Metamucil, Fiberall), which is filled with fiber. Fiber soaks up water in your bowel, making stools larger, softer and easier to pass.

SCRAPES/BURNS

You have a scrape the shape of South America on the side of your leg from laying your bicycle down during a sharp turn on a sandy road. Here's what you do: First wash it with water or a saline solution to clean the dirt out of the wound. Next, smear on an antibiotic ointment that will help prevent infection, then cover the area loosely with a sterile bandage, says Patricia Mertz, research associate professor at the University of Miami School of Medicine in Florida, who specializes in wound healing. In tests of first-aid creams, she found that polymyxin B sulfate (found in Polysporin) healed scrapes fastest, in an average of 8.2 days, followed by neomycin sulfate (found in Neosporin) in 9.2 days. In some cases, says Mertz, neomycin products caused allergic reactions.

If you've suffered a mild burn, such as the kind you get from splattering your skin with hot grease, dab on the same antibiotic first-aid cream to prevent infection. Don't have one handy? Reach for Preparation H, the hemorrhoid treatment; it can slice days off the healing process, says Jerold Z. Kaplan, M.D., medical director of Alta Bates Burn Center in Berkeley, California. Preparation H contains a live yeast derivative that brings more oxygen into the wound site, which in turn speeds healing.

For soothing the sting of a small burn, you can't do better than using a hydrogel, a clear, jellylike bandage made of 96 percent water. One example is Spenco's 2nd Skin moist burn pads. Gels like this promote healing and aid new skin growth.

For sunburn pain, treat your skin to any lotion or ointment containing aloe or 1 percent hydrocortisone, the strongest itch-reliever you can get without a prescription. If large portions of your body are sunburned, an anesthetic spray makes more sense. Try Solarcaine, Lanacane or Bactine Antiseptic/Anesthetic First Aid Liquid or other sprays containing pain-numbing benzocaine, lidocaine, benzyl alcohol or diphenhydramine hydrochloride.

—Jeffrey Csatari

Part 7

LOOKING GOOD

A More Powerful Presence

A new handshake here, the right shoes there, a few other minor alterations—and you're a new man.

••••••••••••••••••

If you're like most men, you're relatively comfortable with your appearance. Maybe you're no Kevin Costner (and judging from his last few films, neither is he), but you dress well, you keep in shape and you don't have too much hair growing out of your ears. And while you may not exactly have to fight them off with a stick, both women and prospective employers seem open to your occasional inquiries.

Every once in a while, though, you look in the mirror and think, "What would life be like if I were more than just good old, lovable me? What would it be like if I were one of those men who walks into a room and commands it?" You know the type. Men respect him, women desire him, small children trust him instinctively. Houseplants bend their leaves in his direction.

Anyone can make an impact if he has enough money or political clout, but there are ways we regular guys, too, can project a persona that commands attention. And we're not talking about visiting Michael Jackson's plastic surgeon. These alterations are simple, reasonable and, for the most part, inexpensive.

GET A GRIP

What's the first thing that happens when you meet someone? Generally, unless he's wielding a knife, you shake hands. That's often the moment when first impressions go awry. You don't want to hand someone a slab of bologna; nor do you want to crush his paw into powder. Your handshake should be naturally firm and steady, the kind of grip that says you're in control but not a brute.

"If there's a trick to the perfect handshake, it's to try to get the webbing between your thumb and forefinger to connect with his," explains Andy Gilman, president of CommCore, a business-communications consulting firm located in New York City and Washington, D.C. "Don't force it in there, but try to give as much hand as possible." Eye contact and a smile are recommended.

To add power to your handshake so it is both firm and natural, strengthen your forearm muscles with a simple exercise called the wrist roll, says Wayne Westcott, Ph.D., national strength-training consultant for the YMCA. Take a foot-long dowel that's about an inch in diameter and drill a hole through the middle. Slip one end of a four-foot rope through the hole and tie it to the dowel, then tie the other end to a five-pound weight. Then grasp each end of the dowel, palms down. Holding your arms straight out in front of you, slowly rotate the dowel toward you with your hands so the rope winds around the dowel and raises the weight. That'll strengthen the muscles on the palm side of the forearm. Once the weight reaches the top, slowly lower it by rotating the dowel away from you. This will work the muscles on the top of the forearm.

A firm shake won't take you too far if your hands feel like fresh oysters. To dry up sweaty palms, try coating them with a roll-on or spray antiperspirant that contains aluminum chloride. (Just wipe off the excess before you venture out.) If the problem persists, consider shock therapy. A $125 device called the Drionic administers very low level electrical current through your palm via a nine-volt battery. The current temporarily plugs up the sweat pores. Contact General Medical Company, Department MNE1, 1935 Armacost Avenue, Los Angeles, CA 90025.

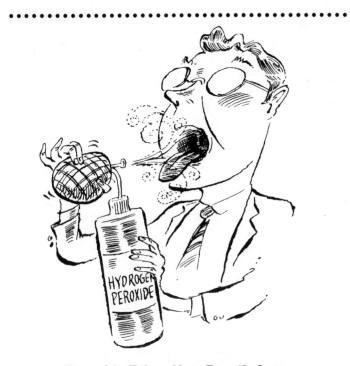

Peroxide Takes Your Breath Away

Dental researchers in England say toothpaste containing hydrogen peroxide is more effective at wiping out bad breath than regular toothpaste. They bravely tested the mouths of ten volunteers and found that brushing with hydrogen peroxide toothpaste reduced odor-causing chemicals in their saliva five times more than did regular toothpaste. Apparently, the peroxide blocks the action of a type of bacteria that causes bad breath odor.

PROJECT YOUR VOICE

For many people, there is nothing more embarrassing than hearing their own voices on audiotape (except maybe watching their golf swing on video). Even a man who thinks his voice projects confidence can be shocked by the sound of his squeaky syllables. That's because when you speak, you hear yourself through the bones in your head, which makes your voice sound deeper than it actually is.

"Our adult voice develops around the age of 12 or 13, but most of us never learn to use it," explains speech therapist Morton Cooper, Ph.D., author of *Winning with Your Voice*. About half of us are still using versions of our childhood voices: nasal, thin and high-pitched. "Watch a talk show," Dr. Cooper says. "Everyone sounds like they're wearing tight pants." Many people, especially men, try to overcome their squeaky voices by talking from the lower throat, in deep, guttural sounds. "That's the way Henry Kissinger talks; he's trying to sound impressive, but mostly he makes you think you're losing your hearing."

So what exactly is your natural adult voice? Say the word "no," forcefully, as if your dog were about to steal a steak off the kitchen table. (If you're reading this on a crowded bus, perhaps this exercise is best saved for later on.) That's your natural voice, Dr. Cooper says—it's deep, strong and assertive and, more important, it will let you speak for long periods of time without going hoarse. With practice, Dr. Cooper says, you can learn to use that commanding voice all the time. Here are some exercises he recommends.

- For starters, make an audiotape of one of your conversations to hear just how you sound to other people. You're likely to be self-conscious if you speak into a tape recorder. So, for more natural results, turn on the recorder the next time you phone a friend. "When you hear yourself played back, all the 'well's and the 'uh's will drive you crazy," says Dr. Cooper.

- When you hum, says Dr. Cooper, you automatically use your natural voice. Hum a few bars of "Happy Birthday," then begin speaking with the same tone you used in humming. Your voice will be more resonant than usual. Since humming at the office is generally not the mark of a man in the fast lane, you can find your best voice using "um-hum." Try inserting it into your speech in place of "ah," "uh," "like," "well" and "you know." Not only will it bring your best voice to the fore, but "um-hum" is also usually received more positively than other little conversational inserts.

■ Breathe more freely. Sit on a chair with one hand on your chest and the other on your midsection. Breathe easily through your nostrils. You should feel your abdomen expand every time you inhale; if instead your chest is moving up and down, you're breathing wrong for speech. "Most men breathe with their upper chest because they're tense or because they've been taught to hold their stomachs in," says Dr. Cooper. The problem with that is it makes you sound nervous and hurried. Breathing with your abdomen allows you to take in more air, which gives your voice a richer, more forceful tone that won't peter out.

■ Find your mantra. Here's an exercise to do when you're certain no one else is home. Remember how forceful the word "no" was when you said it as a command? Use the same tone to say "right," "ready," "go," "do," "be" and "push." Repeat them aloud a number of times. Dr. Cooper says the strength you put into them will stay with you in your daily conversation.

Finally, don't be afraid to change your speaking voice. It won't make you sound phony or intimidating or too much like a bad disk jockey. "That new voice isn't a put-on voice," Dr. Cooper says. "It's your natural one."

STAND UP FOR YOURSELF

You can walk into a meeting with every piece of information you need drilled into your head, but if you slouch, the others will see someone who lacks confidence. Then again, if you concentrate too much on walking erect, not only will you be distracted from the task at hand, you'll appear to have all the spontaneity of Al Gore. Instead, you need a carriage that's linear, yet natural. Stand sideways in front of a full-length mirror. Your hip and shoulder should be in vertical alignment with your ear. If your natural stance looks all out of kilter, take some steps to improve your posture.

One of the main reasons why men develop a slouch is they have too much weight around their midsections. "That forces your back into an arch, which doesn't do your posture any good and is also very bad for your lower back," says Dr. Westcott.

The obvious solution is to trim down, but you also need to strengthen the abdominal muscles, which will keep the pres-

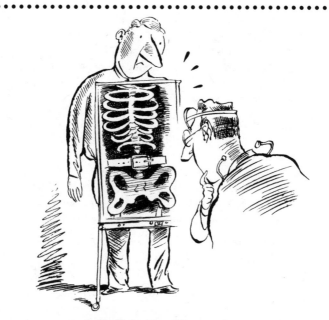

A Belt in the Stomach

A doctor writing in the *Archives of Internal Medicine* says about 25 middle-age men a year come to him complaining of unexplainable stomach cramps, chest pain and heartburn. His diagnosis: Tight Pants syndrome, stomach pain caused by wearing trousers that are too small. Symptoms disappear when the guys accept the gut reality.

sure off your back even if you have some extra fat tissue there. Dr. Westcott recommends crunches, because they put less stress on your lower back than regular sit-ups do. Lie on your back, knees bent and feet flat against the floor. With your fingertips lightly touching your ears, lift your head and shoulders off the floor. At the same time, press your lower back into the floor so that you're reversing the normal curve of the spine. Work up to three sets of ten crunches per day.

A second posture pitfall is tight hamstring muscles, a hazard of sedentary careers. When these large muscles in back of your upper legs tighten, they pull on the pelvis, tilting it down and accentuating the arch in your back, which causes a slouch. To keep hamstrings limber, use what's known as a figure 4 stretch, Dr. Westcott says.

Sit on the floor, right leg out straight and left leg bent at the knee with the bottom of your left foot against your right thigh so your legs form a figure 4. This position will keep stress off your knee and hip, unlike the commonly used hurdler stretch, he says. Now grasp your right toes with your right hand and stretch forward as far as you can. Hold the position for 30 to 60 seconds. If you can't reach your toes, wrap a towel around your foot and grasp the ends of it. Repeat the stretch three times, each time trying to go a little further, then switch legs.

The third thing you can do to improve posture, as well as to prevent back pain, is to strengthen your lower-back muscles. Dr. Westcott recommends using the lower-back exercisers on commercial machines such as Nautilus or Medex. Be sure to consult a trainer at your gym before using one of these machines. If you don't belong to a health club, try this exercise: Lie face down on the floor. Fold your hands under your chin and, using your lower back muscles, gently lift your head and chest off the floor. (You may need someone to hold your legs at first.) Work up to three sets of ten repetitions.

REDRESS YOUR WARDROBE

We know, you've already got more clothes than you can fit into two closets, a dresser and four boxes in the attic. Here are a few tips on how to remake the way you dress without actually buying anything.

■ Worry about the details. They matter most. "When someone comes to me and wants to enhance his style, one of the first things I look at is his shoes. If they're not shined, it's a dead giveaway that he's in need of a style adjustment," says Warren Christopher, a New York City–based image consultant. And while men notice shoes, women seem to notice socks. Toss the plain blacks and blues and opt for subtle stripes, checks and other patterns.

Socks should always reach to at least mid-calf—no showing off patches of hairy leg every time you sit down. Another simple tip that can make a big difference: Keep a steamer and a lint brush at home, and go over jackets and pants before you put them on. What good is a $500 suit if it's got fuzz from your son's teddy bear clinging to the sleeves?

■ Adopt a trademark. George Will has his bow ties; George Burns has his cigars. Perhaps in between is something less nerdy and more healthful that might appeal to you. "A 'signature' is a good way to personalize a wardrobe," says G. Bruce Boyer, fashion writer and author of *Eminently Suitable*. "I have one myself; I always wear brown shoes. It is affected, but as affectations go, it's a mild one." We're not recommending that you start sporting a monocle or a Mohawk. But a little detail—pocket squares, say, or tie clips—can help you create your own personal style.

If you do decide that a trip to the men's department is called for, keep in mind these two key rules: Buy for style, not fashion. In other words, if double-breasted suits are big one year, but they don't look great on you, don't buy one just to be hip. You won't be. Secondly "buy fewer clothes, but buy better clothes," says Boyer. A classic suit will not go out of style, and if it's well-made, it'll last you many years.

Although President Clinton may be changing things with his populist Timex Ironman Triathlon, a good watch can also make a strong statement about you. Don't go for anything clunky or flashy (and please don't even think about trying to get away with one of those sidewalk Rolexes). Buy the best understated gold watch you can afford, and if it has a leather band, replace it as soon as it starts to show signs of wear.

REDO YOUR "DO"

One of the quickest ways to remake your image is to get a new haircut. It's also one of the quickest ways to look like a fool. Remember the '70s? But if Sal down on Hanover Street has been cutting your hair the same way since before they invented electric razors, maybe it's time for a change. If you trust your stylist, go ahead and ask for suggestions. If you're looking for a new barber, ask for a recommendation from a friend with an admirable cut, but make sure he has a hair type similar to yours.

Another important consideration is finding a haircutter who's knowledgeable about men's hair. When you call for an appointment at a new place, ask if they do a lot of men's cuts. Better yet, ask if they color men's hair. "Coloring a man's hair is more exacting than doing a woman's," says Carmine Minardi, co-owner of Minardi-Minardi Salon in New York City. A salon that does is probably very accustomed to taking care of men. Not that *you* want your hair colored, of course.

When you get to the barber's, the first thing you need to discuss is what image you want to project. Yes, we all want to look healthy, wealthy and brimming with sex appeal. But if you've just quit your job and are flying to Tahiti to become a painter, your hairstyle goals are a little different from those of the assistant junior trainee who wants to look mature enough to handle his position. Here are some general rules.

- Small man, short hair. Long hair hides the neck and shoulders and can make a man with a slight frame look even smaller. Instead, you want a somewhat short haircut with a little lift on top to add height and a little length behind the ears to give a vertical frame to the face.

- Big men can't neck. Generally, a bigger man can wear bigger hair, but even if he likes it short, he should leave a little length in the back to cover the hairline at the nape of the neck. If that area is cut close, it can throw the head and neck out of proportion and make them look small in comparison to the broad shoulders.

- Go soft on baby faces. Men with toned faces and chis-eled features can look great with short hair, but those of us who are more chubby of cheek will usually want more mane.

GET PEARL WISDOM

If you have crooked teeth, braces are still an option, and the newer braces are more discreet—no more metal-mouth jokes. Laminates, which are thin layers of porcelain perma-nently bonded to teeth, have dramatically changed the extent to which dentists can alter our looks. Not only can they make teeth straighter-looking, but they can also make you look younger, more assertive, even more masculine. "In two visits we can change the image that a person projects," asserts Irwin Smigel, D.D.S., president of the American Society for Dental Aesthetics. Here are some of the qualities that your dentist may be able to impart.

- Youthfulness. "Yellowish teeth can age you," says Dr. Smigel, because as we age, the outer enamel of our teeth wears down, revealing the yellowish layer under-neath. Porcelain laminates not only whiten your chom-pers—they can also make the teeth longer. Added length will help disguise your true age.

- Improved social standing. "There is a definite socio-economic stigma to crooked or yellow teeth," Dr. Smigel claims. "There is the perception that this person can't afford to take care of his teeth."

- An assertive nature. "Let's say a guy applies for a job at a company where they want someone who is aggres-sive," Dr. Smigel hypothesizes. "They may get the im-pression that he is a go-getter simply from the strength conveyed by his eye teeth." (These are the teeth that look like fangs in bad vampire movies.) By enlarging those and the neighboring teeth and honing the tips just a bit, a dentist can give you a more assertive image.

- A more masculine look. "Small, delicate teeth are a feminine trait," says Dr. Smigel, as are smooth teeth. He makes individuals more masculine-looking by enlarging some of the teeth, most importantly the incisors (the four top front teeth), and providing a coarser texture.

ADVERTISE YOUR SELF-CONFIDENCE

You want people to see you as confident, in control and self-assured. You don't want them to see some swaggering jerk who's so full of himself that he makes Rush Limbaugh look like Mahatma Gandhi. "Balance is the most important part of making a good impression," says Gilman.

For example, eye contact is still the test of honesty in this country, Gilman says. But if you hold someone's gaze too long, or try not to blink, you give the appearance that you're trying to intimidate him. "Think of eye contact as a game of pitch and catch. As I say something to you, I'm throwing this metaphorical ball and watching for a sign that you've caught it." Once you receive that sign—a blink, a nod or an approving murmur—you're free to move your gaze or go on to the next point.

Your stance is also very telling, says Gilman. Here are four common mistakes.

- Slouching can say that you are intimidated, or that you are uninterested in what others have to say. You should try to keep your weight on the balls of your feet. "That position will give you more energy; you should feel capable of moving in any direction," Gilman says.

- Swaying intimates that you are nervous—not the impression you want to give on a job interview or on a first date. If you tend to sway, try putting one foot slightly in front of the other, or opening or closing your stance. This will hold you steady.

- Jangling your keys can really irritate the people you're talking to. If you tend to keep your hands in your pockets, keep other things out of them.

- When you sit, sit back in the seat, but don't rest your back against the backrest, which can lead to slouching. Put one foot slightly in front of the other; it naturally forces your hips forward and makes you look involved.

—Stephen Perrine

Grooming by the Rules

Have a question about grooming? Chances are it's among these top ten.

• • • • • • • • • • • • • • • • • •

Some guys like to play by the rules, and some guys like to break the rules, but all guys at least want to know what the rules are. Even men who've never driven 55 in their lives still like the speed limits to be clearly marked.

But when it comes to clothes and grooming, the rules get pretty hazy. That's because sharing *fashion secrets* ranks low on the male conversation agenda. And for most of us, being on the cutting edge style-wise isn't exactly a priority. But, as with all rules, the consequences of breaking them (a sloppy image) can be costly. We asked top image consultants about the style questions they hear most often and their simple rules for looking sharp.

1. How far should my tie come down?

Your tie should come to a point just below your belt buckle, says Peter Fressola, director of communications for Benetton and formerly men's fashion director for Bloomingdale's. The tie-length rule is founded on the reasoning that the tie should cover all the buttons of the shirt but not be so long that it curls up in your lap like a Chihuahua when you're sitting.

If you find yourself spending extra time in the morning tying and retying it to get it the right length, try a quick midpoint check. Begin to tie your regular knot, but stop just before the point where you'd pull the front of the tie through the last loop. Instead let the long end of the tie drape *over* the loop so it hangs down freely. (It should reach below your belt, since you haven't tightened the knot yet.) Now take the knot in your left hand and lift it so it just touches the base of your throat. This is where the knot will end up when you're done, and if the bottom of the tie now falls at your belt buckle, you're on target and should complete the knot. If it doesn't, loosen the knot and adjust it accordingly.

2. How long should my sideburns be, and how should I trim them?

Start with the middle of the ear—that's a sensible, 1990s

place for your sideburns to fall. If you have an especially wide face, cheat down a quarter-inch to de-emphasize the shape, but don't go below the point where the bottom of the ear joins the face. If your face is long and lean, cheat up a little. Don't make the mistake of shaving your sideburns off altogether. This unsober look should only be sported by those too young to purchase alcohol.

To trim them, start by combing the sideburns back toward your ears; then snip any hairs that extend back beyond the sideburn. To be sure your sideburns are equal, if you're right handed, trim the left one first. Use that as your guideline and trim the right one to match. This will compensate for the natural tendency to trim the nondominant side shorter because of the difference in the reach to that side.

3. Should my belt match my shoes?

"Matching isn't critical," says Fressola, "but common sense is." Your shoes and belt should always be in the same color family—black or gray belts with black shoes, for example, and brown belts with brown shoes. Not just color but shape needs to be considered here: Dress shoes call for an elegant slim belt and casual shoes a wider one. An egregious mismatch only draws the eye to the waist, where most of us can ill afford close scrutiny.

4. My company has started "casual Fridays." How casual should I dress?

"Dress as you would if you were having guests over for a nice, informal dinner," recommends G. Bruce Boyer, fashion writer and author of *Eminently Suitable*. "That means perhaps a pair of khakis, a nice button-down shirt and a sports jacket or sweater." Remember that this is casual business attire, not clothes you'd throw on to rake leaves.

Appropriate footwear depends on how people in your office dress the rest of the week, but you're safest with a casual lace-up or loafer, or even a boat shoe if you're feeling sporty.

5. Should my pants have cuffs?

Many people will tell you that if you're under 5-foot-10, you should avoid them because they break the vertical line of the pants and make you look shorter. "That's a myth," says Boyer. "Cuffs are stylish and have been for 20 years, and there's no reason a shorter man shouldn't wear them."

"A lot of times it depends on the weight of the fabric," of-

fers Warren Christopher, a New York City–based image consultant. Summer-weight fabrics like cotton, linen or silk may
look better with a cuff, because its extra weight holds down
and smoothes the line of the pants legs. But he recommends
against cuffing very thick fabrics—wide-wale corduroys, for
example.

6. Where's the best place to apply cologne?

Anywhere you can take your pulse. Behind your ears, on
your wrist or at the base of your throat are all good choices,
says Lois Mander, assistant vice-president of Ralph Lauren Fragrances. The reasoning? The body's heat rises to the skin's
surface most easily at these pulse points, activating the fragrance more quickly. Another theory holds that since fragrance rises with body heat, you should splash a small amount
of scent on the chest and abdomen. It will slowly rise throughout the day, creating a time-release effect. Either method is
fine, as long as you abide by the one overriding principle of
colognes: just a little, please, for everyone's sake.

**7. I'm 5-foot-7. What are the best tactics for looking
taller?**

To create the illusion of height, you have to accentuate the
body's vertical lines. There are a number of ways to do this.

- Wear pinstripe suits that draw an unbroken line from
head to foot. Conversely, stay away from particularly
large plaids, since the horizontals break that line.

- Use suspenders to lengthen the body. Again, to create vertical lines. Avoid wide belts, which cut the line in
two.

- Wear pants with a high waist. This makes the legs appear longer. Your pants should always sit over your
hips, says Boyer.

- Don't shorten your legs with a long jacket. A common
mistake shorter men make is to wear a regular-cut
jacket. A short man's jacket should end where the buttocks meet the legs—about an inch shorter than normal—to make the legs appear longer. Better men's
stores carry suits and blazers in short, regular and long.

8. What type of shirt collar should I wear?

While there are no hard-and-fast rules, such as which type to wear for business or for a night out, your choice of collar should depend on a couple variables, like the shape of your face and the way you tie your tie.

Round face? Go with pointed collars or button-downs,

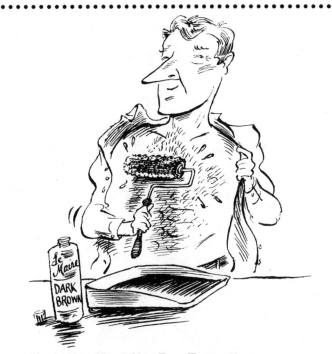

Next Up: Pec Toupees

A little Grecian Formula might disguise your age at the office, but take off your shirt at the beach and your graying chest hair gives you away. What to do? A new trend from California (where else?) is to darken gray chest hair with mix-to-match vegetable dyes. "Paint it on, leave it for 20 minutes and for the next six weeks the men look 20 years younger," says Le Maire (that's her full name, folks) of Le Maire/Hair in Los Angeles. Ask for the treatment at your haircutter's, and for goodness sake, don't tell them we sent you. Prices range from $25 to $75.

both of which will help add length to your chin. Square face, sharp jaw? Wear a collar with rounded tips, or tab or pin collars, which encircle the tie knot and create a softer angle. A long, thin face? Round it off by wearing spread collars. A spread collar is also a good choice if you're developing jowls. (Try to find a picture of Ronald Reagan *not* wearing one.)

If you prefer to tie your tie in stout knots, like half-Windsors, go with spread collars. If you like small, tight knots, like four-in-hands, go with long points.

9. I need a basic business shoe. What's my best bet?

Maybe our fathers drilled this advice into us, but many men reflexively select wingtips for business attire. But wingtips look clunky except when worn with a classic American square-cut suit. For more versatility, you need something a little more sleek. "If you have to get by with one shoe, make it a plain black cap-toe oxford," says Boyer. "It's *the* classic business shoe." Your second choice should be the same thing, only in dark brown, he says.

By the way, if you happen to have big feet—size 11 or bigger—stay away from those flashy Italian shoes you saw in that fashion magazine. They elongate the foot, making you look like you're ready for scuba lessons, not business dealings.

10. How can I get this mustard stain off my shirt in time for my two o'clock meeting?

Here are a few universal guidelines. Act fast and blot the stain—rubbing just pushes it deeper into the fabric. Use detergent, not soap. Your waiter may be able to get you a dollop of the stuff from the kitchen. Also, ask him for some club soda; it's better than plain water in lifting a stain out.

By the way, if you're unfortunate enough to get lipstick on your collar and it's not your wife's shade, try this trick: Place a piece of masking tape on the stain, then yank it off. If that doesn't work, put the tape over your chest hair and do the same thing—maybe then you'll wise up.

—Jack Bettridge

Thinning Hair Cuts

*If heredity left you light-headed, how you cut and style
your hair can make a big difference.*

●●●●●●●●●●●●●●●●●●●

Remember the day your dad grunted and mumbled his
way through an unsophisticated rendition of "the birds and the
bees"? He might not have made it all clear. He might not even
have gotten it all right. And he probably left out one important
issue: "Son, let's talk about balding."

Does that sound farfetched? It shouldn't. Hair loss is as
much a part of being a man as erections and razor burn. Yet
most of us are pretty much left to discover the consequences of
aging on our own. And we're often too late to concede that the
locks we used to feel blowin' in the wind have become as
sparse as, say, hit songs from Bob Dylan.

And therein lies the first mistake: You're not going to get
a haircut that makes the most of what you have unless you can
utter the "B" word to your barber. If you don't feel comfortable
asking him about it, he won't feel comfortable telling you when
your favorite hairstyle is showing more skin than it should. Ask
for an honest assessment of the problem and exactly what he
plans to do about it.

LESS IS ALWAYS MORE

The almost universal rule in dealing with thinning hair is,
less is more. When in doubt, cut. "If the hair is kept shorter, it
actually appears to be fuller," says Anthony Palladino, owner of
Anthony Palladino at the Beverly Hilton barber shop, whose
scissors shear the heads of such sparse-topped media icons as
Jack Nicholson and Bruce Willis. He points out that Willis's all-
around short cut makes his hair look more evenly placed,
when in reality it is concentrated in the back and on the sides.
If Willis tried to grow his hair out, it would bunch together and
the bunches would separate, showing wide expanses of
scalp—and probably leaving Demi Moore up for grabs.

On the other hand, Jack Nicholson purposely grows what

little hair he has long and slicks it back. It works for him, except perhaps on windy days. "It can look wild," says Palladino, "but then again, that's Jack." Since most industries discourage their employees from looking like crazy people, you might want to think twice about emulating Nicholson's hairstyle.

A skilled pair of scissors can also help when hair is thinning only in certain areas. For instance, for many of us, the first indication that all is not as it once was is an obvious thinning in the front: Your hairline is the same as it was in college—it's just limited to a few inches in the center of your forehead. At the temples, the hairline is creeping back like a once green and fertile lawn drying in the August sun. Minimize this condition, called a widow's peak, by trimming the forward part short, while letting the hair at your temples grow longer. Compare *Dirty Harry*–era Clint Eastwood with his *Unforgiven* coif for an idea of how effectively this technique can minimize a receding hairline. An exaggerated version of this cut is called a Caesar, in which the hair is pushed forward to create a false hairline. Kevin Costner in *The Bodyguard* is a good example.

While a receding hairline, properly dealt with, can give a man a certain air of dignity and worldliness, there's not much glamour attached to a bald spot, that circular impression at the crown of the head that can be an especially accursed condition for a shorter man. The strategy here is to keep the back short; long hair in the back of the head will be heavier, pulling down and away from the crown and exposing the balding area. If you still have reasonably thick hair on the top of your head, grow it long and cover the bald spot.

FINE HAIR

If your hair is fine, you're going to have a harder time covering the bald spot—or any spot for that matter. You might want to try what's known in the haircutter's trade as a swell perm, a mild perm that increases hair volume, explains Carmine Minardi, co-owner of Minardi-Minardi Salon in New York City. Such a light perm won't be obvious to others, so you don't have to worry about people at the office pointing at you the next day.

Another salon ploy, if you have dark hair, is to lighten the color a bit. We're not talking about going bleach blonde and looking like an aging Big Kahuna. This is a minor change, with the idea being to cut down on the contrast between the remaining hair and the scalp, thereby making the skin less noticeable. Just make sure you go to a pro; fair-hair men with dark roots do not go over well at board meetings.

When it comes to grooming products, stay away from gels, which can cause sections of hair to stick together and create gorges of empty space that reveal the scalp. Light sprays are better, Palladino says. Wash your hair every day—no, doing so won't make it fall out faster but it will make it look fuller. Don't overcondition your hair; once a week is plenty. Conditioners make hair soft, and while that was fine when you had co-eds running their fingers through your mane, a mature man with thinner hair will find that the softer the hair, the harder it is to style.

THE NOTORIOUS SWEEP

No report on thinning hair would be complete without discussing the metaphysical question most closely associated with baldness: to sweep or not to sweep. You know what we mean. It's tempting to take what's left on the sides and comb it over your dome. Done wrong, this is a disaster, but Palladino says the sweep is an option that should not be ruled out. "The mistake men make is that they let it grow too long," he explains. "Then it will flop around like a toupee." Instead, the hair should reach just across the dome to the hairline on the other side of the head, so it merely *fits* into the open space.

RUGS

A final word: toupees. If you want one, go for it. Just make sure you get a good one that's made from human hair. "Don't try to add too much hair," cautions Palladino. "Bring the toupee in to your barber and have him style your hair around it. You should look like a man your own age who has just started balding," rather than a man wearing a groundhog on his head. Which explains why hairpiece wearer Sean Connery is still an international star . . . and why Burt Reynolds is pitching motor oil.

—*Stephen Perrine*

Fragrant Violations

You'd like to wear cologne, but you don't want to smell like a flower. You need this information.

● ● ● ● ● ● ● ● ● ● ● ● ● ● ● ● ● ● ● ●

It happens to each of us eventually. You're walking through a department store, innocently looking for a wide-screen TV or maybe some new underwear, when you take a wrong turn and find yourself in the cosmetics department.

There must be a way out, you think, but the counters seem to stretch on for miles. You start to panic when you can't find the escalator. Then you see him. He steps from the shadows, a big gift umbrella in one hand and something cocked and loaded in the other. He takes aim.

"Eau de Goopy Toilette?" he says, and before you can answer or make a mad dash for the electronics section, *spritz:* you smell.

The truth is, even without the fragrance goon squad, most of us would rather shop for a sturdy pocketknife and a new remote control than a cologne. We usually leave it up to our significant other to decide what we will smell like. But if you're going to wear an aftershave or cologne—and surveys say that more than 8 out of 10 of us do—there are a couple of big reasons why you should buy it yourself.

First, because of the particular way the stuff interacts with your body chemistry, a given fragrance will smell different on you than it does on anyone else. So you ought to sample it before buying. Second, leave the decision to your wife and the only way she's going to know what cologne to buy is if she smelled it on another man, like maybe that former All-American with the perfect teeth who sits across the hall from her at work. Is that who you want to keep reminding her of?

In the holiday season, manufacturers usually put together gift packages, throwing in luggage or other grooming products cheap. You can often negotiate at the department store and get those packages altered to suit your personal wishes, swapping, say, the bristle brush for an ear-hair trimmer. Another reason to buy during the holidays: Most manufacturers raise their prices in January. Best time of day? The afternoon. Your sense of smell is keener then than in the morning.

PAR-LAY VOUS?

When it comes to negotiating the fragrance counters, don't be put off by all that fancy French jargon. For example, some manufacturers call their fragrance a cologne and others call it an eau de toilette. These are essentially the same thing, says Annette Green, president of the Fragrance Foundation in New York City. If you do see both a cologne and an eau de toilette from the same company, the difference is in the degree of concentration. The scent of the more concentrated one will last longer. How do you know the difference? Go by price, says Green. The more expensive one will carry further into the day. A step lower down the scale are aftershaves, which are formulated to last only a brief time. They generally just give you a quick whiff of fragrance while also having an astringent effect on your face, making it feel cleaner. An aftershave's scent will disappear about midway through the morning commute, but if you use a cologne and an aftershave, make sure they're both the same brand, otherwise the people in your car pool will think they're riding with Sybil. Another important translation: *Pour Homme* or *Per Uomo* means it's for guys.

To know what you're talking about as you flirt with the woman behind the fragrance counter, you'll need to know the different elements that go into men's fragrances. Experts divide them into five subsets.

■ Sportive fragrances are based on citrus, from the oils of limes, lemons and oranges, and spices, like bay, cinnamon and nutmeg. They tend to carry a lighter scent and are good choices for wearing around the office. Often these are easily identified by their names, such as Canoe, Nautica and Polo Crest.

■ Poetic scents contain lavender oil. Don't panic; lavender was the chosen fragrance of cowboys, who bathed in it after cattle drives, so it has a very manly pedigree. Good for day use. Brands include Eternity for Men and Feraud Pour Homme.

- Relaxed scents, such as Bel Ami by Hermes, bear a leathery aroma, which is created from the resin of birch and other trees. To wear in the evenings.

- Sophisticated fragrances such as Boucheron or Guess Men take their essences from woody scents like cedar and sandalwood and forest fragrances like moss. For a night out at the local brasserie.

- Erotic colognes tend to be the most flowery, since they are generally a blend of exotic flowers and herbs. One example is Joop! Homme. We don't think we have to tell you what to wear this for.

● ●

Scar Tactics

Every guy has a scar or three, reminders of more rambunctious days. No big deal. They're part of life. But if your face is cratered with acne or chicken-pox scars that bother you or if a scar links you to a mishap you'd like to forget (that time you played Night of the Crash Test Dummies), plastic surgeons are waiting in the wings, eager to help. These are the main scar-repair options, according to Richard A. Marfuggi, M.D., a Manhattan plastic surgeon.

Steroids. Injected directly into certain scars, steroids can reduce itching and redness, flatten the scar and soften the skin.

Surgical revision. The scar is cut out and the wound is cleanly restitched with internal and external sutures.

Z-plasty or W-plasty. A scar that crosses the natural creases of the body, such as the lines extending from your nose to the corners of your mouth when you smile, can be made less noticeable by surgically changing the scar's direction. First, the old scar is cut away, then flaps are made on each side of the wound and rotated to cover it, creating a new scar in a different direction.

Dermabrasion. For bad acne scarring, a wire brush is used to remove the top layer of skin. New skin growing back is smoother, flattening the appearance of the pitted areas.

Chemical peels. Similar to dermabrasion, except the top layer of skin is treated with an acid solution that causes the skin to peel.

Hydroquinine. This chemical can be applied to skin to fade the brown discoloration of a scar.

When you try out a cologne, give it time to dry on your skin before you shell out any money. A connoisseur will search for three distinct levels of aroma from each cologne. The "top note" is what you smell when you first open the bottle. It should tell you immediately what category of fragrance you're dealing with, so if you want something to wear yachting and this smells more like peat moss, don't even try it on.

If you like the first whiff, however, put a drop or two on your skin and test the "body" (or middle note) of the fragrance, which is what it smells like as it dries over the next minute or two. Once the cologne is completely dry, smell it again. This smell is the final note, which is what the cologne is going to leave you smelling like for the next three or four hours. If this all sounds complex, it's supposed to be. Think of it as on a par with tasting a fine wine; there's a bit more subtlety in a good department-store fragrance than in that blue stuff you used to pick up at the drugstore.

GET YOUR MONEY'S WORTH

Okay, so you successfully negotiated the hazards of the fragrance counter and got the stuff home. Here are some things to remember so you get your money's worth from it.

- Cologne can dry your skin, so keep it off your face and any areas that tend to be dry. Fragrance rises, so apply it low, but keep it away from your privates (even if you're feeling lucky tonight—the stuff can sting).

- Less is more, especially if you have oily skin, which tends to hold the scent longer.

- Don't mix cologne with scented deodorants or soaps, unless they come from the same brand line. Too many scents spoil the stew.

- To preserve its intensity, keep it tightly sealed and store it away from heat and light. That means if you like hot showers, keep it out of the bathroom. Any fragrance will lose much of its power after about a year no matter where you store it, so no splashing on that bottle of Hai Karate you bought in 1972.

Is all this purely a vanity issue? Probably, but wearing a scent might do more than just mark you as a well-groomed man. Research is underway at Duke University in Durham, North Carolina, to see if colognes can help middle-age men overcome depression—they've already been found to have some positive impact on older women.

A final safety note: The alcohol content of cologne makes it highly flammable, so be careful with it. Set that table for a romantic dinner, light those candles, then try to spritz on a last bit of cologne, and *whoosh*! An entirely different type of spontaneous combustion than what you were hoping for.

—Stephen Perrine

Part 8

BOD LIKE A ROCK

Fast Muscle

*What good is all that sweat and effort if it doesn't
make you look good in jeans? Here's how to make
sure you get visible results—fast.*

•••••••••••••••••

IF YOU'RE GOING THROUGH all the bother of joining a
health club, fitting workouts into an already impossible
schedule and lugging all those sweaty clothes around in the
backseat of the car, you can't be blamed if you want something to show for it. And fast.

Mainly what you want to show for it are some new,
bulging muscles, correct? Cardiovascular health, stress relief, fewer back problems—those are all fine reasons to exer-

cise, but what good are they if you don't look better in a T-shirt and jeans?

Now that we understand each other, here's a fitness program that will give you results—*visible* results—in only a few weeks.

A study by the YMCA offers proof that you can put on muscle with extraordinary speed. Some subjects who were guided through an intense exercise program for 20 minutes three times a week gained up to 6 pounds of muscle and lost as much as 15 pounds of fat in just seven weeks. "Granted, it was a pretty grueling workout," says Wayne Westcott, Ph.D., the YMCA's national strength-training consultant and *Men's Health* magazine advisor. "But it shows us there are optimum ways to gain muscle quickly." That doesn't mean you have to look forward to a lifetime of hard labor. Once you've put in your seven weeks and attained the level of muscle growth you're looking for, you can afford to downshift a bit—without losing that new physique you worked so hard for. Unlike your golf swing or your marriage, muscles are something you can keep in top shape without constant attention. "As little as one strength-training session a week is all you need to help preserve muscle mass once you've gained it," says Alan Mikesky, Ph.D., associate director of research at the National Institute for Fitness and Sport in Indianapolis.

We asked experts in the field of muscle development for a workout plan that delivers results fast without requiring excessive gym time. No problem, they told us. "An hour of resistance training three times a week should be more than sufficient to see positive results," says Bill Pearl, four-time Mr. Universe and author of *Getting Stronger*. We'll get to the specific exercises below, but first let's take a look at the principles of rapid muscle growth.

●●

Shift Differential

You may get more out of your workout if you schedule it for the afternoon, suggests a study from Japan. Researchers there found that men who exercised on a stationary cycle at three o'clock improved their aerobic fitness significantly more than men who worked out at nine in the morning or eight at night. The scientists theorize that body changes that occur in the afternoon may make exercise more effective at that time.

Take muscles to the limit. To get the speediest growth, you have to push your muscles to the point where you can't do another repetition. This is known as *fatiguing* the muscle, and it requires that you work out with heavy weights, about 70 percent of the maximum you could raise in a single lift. Weight training builds strength by putting strain on the muscles and actually breaking down microscopic muscle fibers. The gains come in the recovery process. As the muscles "heal" from the workout, they rebuild bigger and stronger.

Start off with a full tank. For every hour that you lift weights, your body needs at least 300 to 500 additional calories. You want most of these calories in the form of carbohydrates. "Carbohydrates fuel the workout, so that your protein stores can go straight to muscle building rather than being broken down for fuel," says Georgia Kostas, R.D., nutrition director of the Cooper Clinic in Dallas and author of *The Balancing Act Nutrition and Weight Guide*. High-carbohydrate, low-fat, 500-calorie snacks include a cup of cereal and skim milk, a banana and four tablespoons of raisins; a cup of low-fat yogurt and six fig bars; or a bagel, a pint of grape juice and an apple.

Don't make the common bodybuilder's mistake of thinking you need a lot of extra protein throughout the day. The average American diet delivers more than enough protein anyway. Look to get about 450 calories from protein daily, the amount in a lean quarter-pound hamburger, a large chicken-breast sandwich, a serving of pinto beans and a 16-ounce glass of skim milk.

Limit lifts to two sets. Just because you want to push the muscle to fatigue, that doesn't mean you have to camp out at each weight station. "Doing more than two sets causes the muscle to take longer to recover and could, in the long run, hurt your progress," says Chet Fuhrman, conditioning coordinator for the Pittsburgh Steelers professional football team.

Start heavy, end light. Experts say your first set should be done with the heaviest weight you plan to use. This runs counter to the popular practice of doing your first set with a modest amount of weight and then piling on more weight plates for each succeeding set. Explains Fuhrman: "If you start with a light weight first, you create so much fatigue in the beginning that when it's time for an all-out effort, you don't have anything left." Warm up by going through the motions with very light weight. Then, for your first set, start right in with the heaviest weight you're planning to lift—again roughly 70 percent of the maximum weight you could lift just once. Try for 8 to 12 repetitions. For the second set, decrease the weight 5 to 15 pounds or whatever amount it takes so that you can pump out at least 8 to 12 repetitions before exhausting the muscle.

If you can, count to ten. Exercise physiologists now recommend spending seven to ten seconds lifting the weight and four seconds lowering it. Doing so not only helps keep you from jerking or heaving the weight up, cheating your muscles out of a proper workout, but it also employs more muscle fibers for longer periods of time. In one study, men who spent ten seconds lifting the weight and four seconds bringing it down increased strength 50 percent faster than those following the more conventional practice of lifting in two seconds and lowering in four. Using this technique, you should lower the poundage to between 55 and 65 percent of the maximum weight you could lift just once.

Do your best, then rest. "Rest is as important as weight lifting itself," says Wayne Campbell, Ph.D., of the Noll Laboratory for Human Performance Research at Pennsylvania State University in University Park. After all, it's not during the weight-lifting process, but in the recovery period that muscles start to grow. That rest should be 48 hours long. "If you don't allow at least that much time between sessions, you may actually find yourself getting weaker because your muscle will constantly be in the broken-down phase," says Dr. Campbell. Studies done at McMaster University in Hamilton, Ontario, show that the body's internal muscle-rebuilding process reaches its peak one full day after you put down your last weight and continues well into the next day if not interrupted. Another kind of short-term recovery takes place between sets as your muscles regain enough strength to go on to set number two. And it's critical to rapid gains that you use this time efficiently, giving your muscles just enough rest so you can deliver full effort. According to the experts, within 60 seconds of putting the weight down, your muscles recover nearly 75 percent of their energy, and within two minutes, they recover nearly all of it. For maximum power on your second set, be sure to rest at least 60 seconds for upper-body exercises and the full two minutes for the larger muscles in the legs.

Save your energy for the iron. If fast muscle gain is your primary goal, don't do too much running or other aerobic exercises. "To gain muscle rapidly, it's detrimental to be burning a lot of energy in other activities," says exercise physiologist Gary Hunter, Ph.D. In studies at the University of Massachusetts in Amherst, subjects who lifted weights and then rested posted more than twice the strength gains of another group who lifted weights and then ran two miles.

Drive yourself, then drink. Experts recommend drinking as much as a glass of water *every hour* during the days you train. That's an awful lot of water, but your muscles require it. "Most weight lifters don't hydrate themselves properly," says Dr. Westcott. If you don't, you'll limit your body's ability to grow. Water comprises 75 percent of muscle fiber and is used for everything from muscle contraction to cooling, so proper hydration is vital in generating muscle tissue.

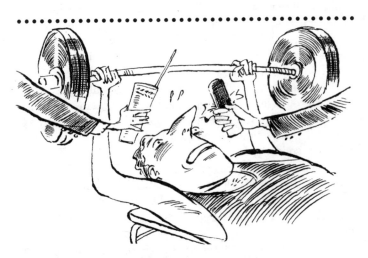

Best Fuel for the Long Run

You're two hours into a workout and you feel your energy waning. You have your choice of one of the carbohydrate-rich sports drinks or sports bars. Which is better? In an Australian study, when six trained athletes consumed equal amounts of each, blood tests showed that sports bars and sports drinks were equally effective in delivering glucose, the blood sugar the muscles use for fuel.

Get in, then get out. Our final note concerns a practical matter: wasted time. At any given health club on any given day, you'll notice that half the people there *aren't* working out. If you really want to save time, don't hang around and compare war stories, don't flex your muscles in the mirror and don't stop at the juice bar for an apple-carrot spritzer. Get into your shorts, get working, then go home. You'll be amazed at how much more economically your valuable exercise minutes are being spent.

THE PROGRAM

To start building muscle fast, you need to perform exercises that call into play not specific muscles but groups of muscles. It's a matter of efficiency. Compound exercises, as these are called, deliver more of a return for your exercise investment. The ultimate example is the squat, which works 256 different muscles in just one motion, making it the ideal lower-body exercise.

For this workout, the demands of efficiency include a short but thorough warm-up. The risk of muscle pulls or strains is higher when you're lifting heavier weights. Get your muscles primed and the joints limber with five minutes of light calisthenics or stationary cycling and some stretching. Then perform the exercises below, designed to hit all of the major muscle groups for balance and body symmetry. Anyone who's not actively lifting weights should stay with very light weights for a full week's time to get back in the swing of things and minimize soreness.

Perform the following exercises two or three times a week. Shoot for two sets of at least 8 repetitions, but no more than 12. If you can do more repetitions, take that as a sign that you should be adding more weight. Raise the stakes in five-pound increments until you're back in the 8- to 12-repetition range.

Squat (works the large muscles of the legs and butt): In a standing position, place a barbell on a squat rack and position yourself in front of the bar. With your legs shoulder-width apart and your feet pointing straight ahead, lift the barbell off the rack. With your chest out and your shoulder blades tucked in, squat down until your thighs are almost parallel to the floor. (You should stop before your thighs are parallel to the floor.) Stand up again.

Bench Press (works upper and lower chest muscles, triceps and front deltoids): Lie on an exercise bench and grip a barbell with your hands slightly more than shoulder-width apart. Lift the bar off the rack. Slowly lower the weight until it just touches your chest lightly. Then press the bar upward above your chest, raising it as high as you can without locking your elbows.

Pulldown (exercises the back muscles, biceps and forearms): For this one, you'll need access to a lat-pulldown machine on a multistation gym. Stand facing the machine. Reach up and grasp the bar with an overhand grip that's four to six inches wider than your shoulders. Next, kneel in front of the machine, letting the resistance of the bar extend your arms above your head. When you're in position, pull the bar down until it touches the back of your neck just above the shoulders. Hold this position for a second, then return it to the starting position.

Military Press (works the shoulders, triceps and upper back): Sitting on an exercise bench, grasp a barbell (or a set of dumbbells) with your hands shoulder-width apart. Press the weight straight overhead, hold for a count of one, then bring it down to rest on the front of your shoulders. Raise the weight again until your arms are almost fully extended. Hold for a beat, then return to the front of your shoulders.

Upright Row (works the upper back and shoulders): Grasp the middle of a barbell with your hands about six inches apart. Standing with your back and head straight, slowly raise the bar to your chin. Hold for a second before returning to the starting position.

Triceps Pushdown (exercises the muscles located in back of the upper arms): While standing, grip the bar attached to a high-pulley cable or lat machine with your hands about six inches apart. With your elbows tucked against your sides,

• •

Hands-Off Training

You may get a better workout on a stair climber if you keep your hands to yourself. Research conducted at the University of Wisconsin-La Crosse suggests that people burn more calories on stair-climbing machines when they swing their arms rather than hold on to the handrails for support.

bring the bar down until it is directly in front of you. With your forearms parallel to the floor (the starting position), push the bar down until your arms are extended straight down, with the bar near your thighs. Don't lock your elbows. Return to the starting position.

Leg Extension (works the quadriceps, located on the tops of the thighs): Sitting in a leg-extension machine with your feet under the footpads, lean back slightly and lift the pads with your feet until your legs are extended. Hold for a second, then return.

Biceps Curl (exercises the muscles on the front of the upper arms): Sitting on the end of an exercise bench, grasp a dumbbell in each hand and let your arms hang to your sides. Curl the weights upward toward your shoulders, hold for a second, and lower them to the starting position.

Leg Curl (works the hamstring muscles, located behind the thighs): Lying face down on a leg-curl machine, tuck the backs of your heels underneath the footpads. Curl the weight upward until your feet are near your buttocks. Hold for a second before returning to the starting position.

Finish your session with two sets of stomach crunches, which work the abdominal muscles, and two sets of pull-ups. Then stretch and cool down with a few minutes of light aerobics.

Follow this program and you'll see your muscles begin to stand up and be counted. Once you've built the body you want, you can stick with the regimen for additional gains or merely maintain it with a once-a-week workout. Regardless of how far you go, you'll have much more confidence in taking off your shirt at the beach next summer—and no one's going to kick sand in your face again.

—*David Zinczenko*

Flab Fighters

In the case of aerobic exercise, a guy likes to know what he stands to lose from his efforts.

• • • • • • • • • • • • • • • • • • •

HERE'S A LITTLE CHART to show you how many pounds you can expect to drop by getting some regular exercise. Just 40 minutes of one of the following activities three days a week will leave you trimmer in less than two months.

The following figures are based on a 176-pound man.

Activity	Calories burned in 40 min.	Total weight lost (lb.)
Basketball	472	3.2
Boxing (sparring)	440	3.0
Cycling (9.4 mph)	320	2.2
Frisbee	320	2.2
Golf	272	1.9
Jogging (7 min./mile)	716	4.9
Jumping rope (80/min.)	524	3.6
Scuba diving	568	3.9
Softball	220	1.5
Stair climbing	540	3.7
Swimming (slow crawl)	408	2.8
Tennis	460	3.2
Volleyball	472	3.2
Walking (4 mph)	312	2.1

Plateau Busters

To learn anything—whether a better golf swing or a new job skill—requires not just forward progress but also the occasional step backward.

●●●●●●●●●●●●●●●●●●

YOU KNOW ABOUT THE LAW that says you can be arrested for impersonating a male if you don't invest at least 21 percent of your attention in getting better at something—preferably work, sports, physical conditioning, playing electric guitar or earning the approval of women (not necessarily in that order). Improving yourself as a mate, father or civic activist will also do, thanks partly to the spillover from one area to others.

And you may have noticed a sure way to run afoul of that law: Between jumps in performance, you hit a long stretch where you see scant results from all your effort, and you're tempted to quit outright or at least slack off trying to improve.

Let's say you attack a project—to build muscle mass, smoothen your golf swing, eat less fat, make swifter decisions, whatever. You adopt some new moves, and after a while you have a spurt of progress. Aha, the breakthrough; from here on it's a steady climb to mastery. But what is this? The climb levels off—worse yet, when you add a new move to the ones you've just become adept in, it actually dips down. You keep making the moves, but the payoffs come farther apart. The excitement wanes. You feel something akin to the workout stagnation that fitness trainers often see. You haven't hit anything as tidy as a wall; more like a plateau with no peaks ahead.

I might be a decent tennis player by now if I hadn't been fed up with my serve resisting betterment in the summer I was 13. (And a passable cellist, come to think of it, if I'd stuck with the practice. And maybe I'd have understood chemistry if... but that's another story.)

We know something that most 13-year-olds don't. Performance plateaus are not a penalty for ineptitude, impatience or excess machismo. They're the law—a real one this time. The brain-muscle-gland setup of a human being requires plateaus in learning and training of any kind.

Experienced athletes program "muscle memory" by repeating a movement over and over, no matter how flat and unprofitable the practice seems. Everyone knows that. Athletes know a plateau is no obstacle at all, as an eminent investigator of human performance—my friend and colleague George Leonard, author of *The Ultimate Athlete*, a high-ranking black belt and teacher of aikido—points out. To the contrary, it is an essential stage in any journey toward new levels of competence.

MASTERY

"There's really no way around it," Leonard writes in his most recent book, *Mastery*. "Learning any new skill involves relatively brief spurts of progress, each of which is followed by a slight decline to a plateau somewhat higher, in most cases, than that which preceded it." Of course you practice, but you also have to be willing to spend most of your time on a plateau, to keep practicing even when you seem to be getting nowhere.

This is not bad news, Leonard makes clear. All the while you're on a plateau, your system is accumulating information it will use for the next upward leap. Having a grasp of what's happening inside you can open up one of the great secrets of true mastery: the ability to practice primarily for the sake of the practice itself. Learning to love the plateau.

To check this out with a guy wiping sweat off his face, I went over to the Mt. Tam Racquet Club in Larkspur, California, and met Derek Scott. An athletic man of 45 who played ice hockey as a teenager and football and rugby in college, Scott found himself challenged by one plateau after another when he first took up tennis five years ago.

Lessons started with Scott in a fixed position and a coach feeding him balls, one after another, to hit back: forehand forehand forehand, backhand backhand backhand, forehand, backhand, dozens in a row. The Mt. Tam tennis pro who introduced us, David Kowalski, won't move students beyond the basic ground strokes until he sees real consistency like hitting the ball in the middle of the racket, over the net and in the court every time. Scott moved quickly to that level.

"I thought I was doing pretty well," he said. "Then the pro started to rally with me [i.e., hit back each ball Scott hit]. Suddenly, my level dropped."

He felt he had lost some of what he had gained, "because, instead of having a nice fat ball fed right to me, now I had to chase it around, it had a different spin . . ." He was learning there's more to the game than solid strokes; there's also *moving to the ball* to make the stroke. So he got good at that, and had another spurt of progress. Then he moved up to shot placement—cross court, down the line—and again his competence dipped.

Scott stayed with the program, reminding himself, "This is a game, I'm having fun, and I'm paying this person to tell me how to get better."

Again he got good. "Then I went out and played somebody else who was learning, and I found I couldn't do it at all. His shots weren't well-directed, and he wasn't being paid by me to make me look good. I dropped again."

RIDE THE LEARNING CURVE

Scott was on a classic learning curve. Kowalski breaks it down into four stages.

1. Unconscious incompetence. You're unaware of what you're doing wrong.

2. Conscious incompetence. You become aware, usually through coaching, of what it looks like to do it right.

3. The hardest part. You train muscle memory, paying attention to the technique and repeating it. "This is the plateau," Kowalski acknowledges. "You can practice day in and day out for a month and see no significant improvement. Then all of a sudden, you've got the best shot of your life. Everything drops into place."

4. Unconscious competence. You become unaware again—doing it right without having to think about it.

To portray the mechanism behind the spurt-plateau rhythm, Leonard cites the pioneering brain research of Karl Pribram, M.D., who retired from Stanford University after 30 years and heads the Center for Brain Research and Informational Sciences at Radford University in Virginia.

The nucleus of what goes on when you learn something is

an *automatic processing system* that works at a level deeper than conscious thought. It consists of circuits in the brain that connect sensory input (seeing the flight of the ball, for example) with motor output (raising your racket to strike the ball). The motor output includes what your muscles do and, to some extent, what your endocrine glands do to keep you alert but not too tense. "Lots of feedback loops," Dr. Pribram explains. This is the system you use to do many things like lift weights, return a serve or drive a car and talk at the same time without worrying about exactly how you do them.

When you start to learn a new skill, you have to replace old automatic patterns with new ones. This requires paying attention. "You need a lot more brain," Dr. Pribram said. What happens as you learn something new is that an *effort system*, centered at the base of the brain, triggers a set of *cognitive systems*, those you use for controlled thinking. The cognitive systems operate on the automatic processing system long enough to reprogram it, a short time or long time, depending on the individual and the complexity of the task. When the reprogramming is done, the cognitive systems withdraw, and you're back on automatic. And ready to start the process again.

In this light, Leonard sums up, you can see that the upward spurts on your learning curve are by no means the only times significant things are happening. The next time you feel stranded on a plateau, think of your cognitive systems purring along behind the scenes, reprogramming your automatic processing system to a new task, and remember there's going to be a moment when they withdraw. "This means," Leonard says, "you can perform the task without making a special ef-

• •

Running at the Equator

If experience were a good teacher, we'd have to say that the fat located in a potbelly is the most stubborn. But a study from Washington University in St. Louis suggests that all it takes to shrink this recalcitrant zone is hard work. Men in this study walked or ran for an average of 45 minutes four times a week at a rather good clip: 80 percent of their maximal heart rates. Over 9 to 12 months, they lost an average of 3.7 percent of their body fat, mostly from the midriff.

fort to think of its separate parts. At this point, there's an apparent spurt of learning. But this learning has been going on all along."

So here is science reinforcing philosophy, and both of them reinforcing the perennial wisdom: Follow a practice for its own sake. Learn to love the plateau.

GO FOR THE BURN-IN

Masterful athletes appreciate the plateau for what it is—a time when they're burning in new nerve pathways, accumulating strength, getting ready for the eventual big moment—and simultaneously as a real satisfaction in its own right. That knowledge isn't reserved for just a gifted few. Any of us can approach nutrition, exercise patterns and other health habits as a practice, in the sense of doing a simple routine over and over, but also in the sense of being on a journey of discovery. It's this journey that constitutes a master's path, transforming good habits into the kind of discipline that shapes a life.

—John Poppy

The Month-by-Month Workout

Looking for a comprehensive program to make you stronger without spending long hours in the gym? You've found it.

• • • • • • • • • • • • • • • • • •

NEW YEAR'S DAY. You awaken to a living room that resembles a fraternity house during hell week: champagne bottles, confetti and funny hats litter the tables; a crusty twig of mistletoe dangles from the light fixture and a big green fire hazard covered with tinsel stands by the hearth. Your own physical status isn't much better. One look in the mirror at the gut you developed over the last month and you make an immediate pledge. But there's not a guy in your neighborhood who isn't making the same resolution: *This year I'm going to get in shape and stay in shape.* All well and good, except for one sticking point. Study after study shows that about 50 percent of men drop out of their workout programs in the first six months, and fewer still are getting to the gym regularly by year's end. Almost everyone who's taken up exercise has at some point dropped out—you probably have, too. Why is a workout routine so hard to stick to? Lots of reasons: lack of progress, lack of time or simply having more pressing things to do with your off-hours. But the most important reason men drop out of their exercise programs is that they get bored with them, says Doug Lentz, owner and manager of the Chambersburg Sports Medicine and Rehabilitation Center in Pennsylvania and strength coach for Olympic marathoner Steve Spence.

What you need is a comprehensive exercise program that will show results without keeping you in the gym for hours a day, and one that's varied enough that you get a good workout without feeling bored.

How's that for a resolution?

The key to making an exercise program work is to set goals for yourself. What you need is to combine both the big picture ("I want to lose some weight and build some muscle, so I can take my shirt off at the beach this summer.") and the little picture ("I want to move up one level on the StairMaster next week."). So we've arranged our program in two ways: with month-to-month goals that will help you see your progress, and with seasonal goals that will keep you in touch with just what you're trying to accomplish here.

First, a reality check. You are not idly rich. You do not have endless stretches of time to spend in trendy health spas, chasing the latest exercise fads. You have a job, friends, family, hobbies and a faulty transmission that needs to be attended to. You simply can't stick to some Herculean exercise program. Fortunately, you don't have to, says Bill Pearl, a four-time Mr. Universe and author of *Getting Stronger.* A simple three-day-a-week routine that combines weight training and aerobics is all you need to build muscle, trim off fat and start feeling fitter.

THE CORE WORKOUT

Five minutes of warm-up. Brisk walking, jogging in place, easy stationary biking, whatever. Follow this with a few minutes of light stretching.

Fifteen minutes of aerobic activity. You can do the same exercise you did for your warm-up, or you can do something completely different.

Thirty minutes of weight lifting. You'll be doing one to two sets of eight to ten repetitions, focusing on the major muscle groups, using the exercise stations described below. Rest 60 to 90 seconds between sets.

Five minutes of cooldown. Do two sets of sit-ups or crunches and some light stretching, concentrating on muscles that feel tight.

EXERCISE STATIONS

Squat (builds overall leg strength): In a standing position, grasp a barbell with your hands slightly wider than shoulder-width apart (use a squat rack and spotter for safety). Rest the bar behind your head and across your shoulders. Keeping your hands on the bar, squat down as if about to sit on a chair, but stop before your thighs are parallel to the floor. Return to the upright position. Repeat. *Alternative*: seated leg press.

Bench Press (works upper and lower chest and triceps): Lying on an exercise bench with your knees bent so your feet are flat on the floor, grab a barbell with your hands slightly wider than shoulder-width apart. Lift the bar off the rack, then slowly lower it to your chest. Press the weight up until your arms are extended, but stop before your elbows are locked. Hold for a count of two, then lower and repeat. *Alternative*: dumbbell fly.

Leg Extension (develops quadriceps or upper leg muscles): Sit in a leg-exercise resistance machine with your feet under the footpads and your back straight. Raise the weight stack until your legs are fully extended, but stop before your knees lock. Hold for a second, then return to the starting position. *Alternative*: lunge.

Leg Curl (works hamstrings): Lying face down on a leg-curl machine, place your feet under the footpads. Bending your knees, raise your calves until the footpads are almost touching the backs of your thighs. Return to the starting position and *Alternative*: standing leg curl.

Pulldown (builds back muscles, biceps and forearms): Reach up and take an overhand grip on the bar of a lat-pulldown machine, with your hands four to six inches wider than your shoulders. Sit down in the machine, placing your knees beneath the restraint pads. Pull the bar down until it touches the top of your chest. Hold one second, then return slowly to the starting position. *Alternative*: dumbbell row, chinup.

Military Press (strengthens shoulders, triceps and upper back): Sitting on an exercise bench, feet flat on the floor, grasp a barbell with your hands slightly wider than shoulder-width apart. Lift the weight over your head. Then slowly lower the bar in front of you until it's even with your chin. Raise the weight again until your arms are almost fully extended. Hold for a beat, then return to the starting position. *Alternative*: dumbbell shoulder press.

Triceps Pushdown (works the triceps and shoulder muscles): Stand in front of the lat-pulldown machine and grip the bar attached to a high-pulley cable, hands about six inches apart. With your elbows tucked against your sides, bring the bar down until your forearms are parallel to the floor (the starting position). Now extend your arms until the bar is near your thighs. Return to the starting position, then repeat. *Alternative*: two-handed triceps extension, dip, triceps kickback.

Biceps Curl (isolates the biceps): Stand and hold a barbell with an underhand grip so that your arms are extended naturally and the bar touches your thighs. With elbows tucked against your sides, slowly bring the bar up to your chest. Hold, then slowly lower the weight to the starting position. *Alternative*: seated dumbbell curl.

Here's your basic plan: Three days a week, with at least one day's rest between sessions and follow the Core Workout on page 224. Then check out our guide to keeping your workout fun and effective all year long.

WINTER: IN LIKE A LION, OUT LIKE A LEANER, TRIMMER LION

Consider the first eight weeks as time to get the engine revved. This means, above all, taking it slowly. "Most people ruin a good plan because they jump out of the starting gate too quickly and make their workouts grueling," says Pearl. "Your attitude is as important as the routines themselves. Try to have fun, or else you won't want to come back."

What this means is worrying about consistency, not intensity. If you spend ten minutes trying to figure out the StairMaster instead of hammering your way through the hardest level, that's fine. Just get comfortable with the machine and with your routine, and realize that it takes time to build skills. By the time you start to smell the first whiff of spring in the air, you will have made enough progress to feel like a serious exerciser—or at least like someone who doesn't spend too much time on the sofa with a can of Pringles.

January

The Goal: To get to the gym three times a week. That's it. But it's trickier than it seems.

The Program: Start slowly, giving your body time to get

• •

Pedaling under the Influence

If you drink, don't drive. Your bicycle, that is. A report on bicycling injuries published by the Johns Hopkins Injury Prevention Center found that men are nearly 2½ times more likely to die on their bikes than are women. The study also indicated that alcohol plays a clear role in a significant number of fatal bicycle accidents. Of the 2,723 bikers 15 or older killed from 1987 to 1991, two-thirds were tested for alcohol and more than one-third had been drinking. The majority of men who tested positive had blood-alcohol concentrations over 0.10 percent, which is considered too high for safely operating a vehicle—any vehicle—in most states.

accustomed to your routine and start to build muscle and endurance and begin melting fat. Follow the instructions for the Core Workout on page 224, staying at less than 60 percent of your maximum heart rate during the aerobic portion of your workout. To figure out your maximum heart rate, subtract your current age from 220. For example, let's say you're 36. Your maximum heart rate is 184, so 60 percent of that is 110 beats per minute. (Plenty of exercise machines will run this little computation for you.)

The rule of thumb for January is to show up. If you don't get all the exercises done, if you don't feel like you're putting in the effort you should, if you're feeling tired or hassled, that's okay. At least get to the gym three days a week and do what you can.

It doesn't seem too complicated, but there are pitfalls waiting for you right from the beginning. If you haven't been exercising regularly, the most likely one is muscle soreness. Not only will it leave you feeling stiff the next day, it will also hamper your willingness to get back to the gym and your rate of improvement once you do get there. Pearl recommends that for the first month of your weight-training workout, you lift no more than 65 to 70 percent of your maximum weight. Your maximum is the most weight you could lift in a single repetition. For example, if you are capable of bench-pressing 150 pounds once, then begin your bench-press sets with 105 pounds on the bar.

February

The Goal: To maintain your routine and customize it according to your individual goals and abilities.

The Program: Using the Core Workout on page 224 as a guide, substitute alternative exercises that seem to work better for you.

You can buy any number of workout books or tapes by the fitness guru of the moment, who's going to tell you how to get abs of steel or buns of steel or thumbs of steel or whatever. The problem with many of these one-size-fits-all programs is that every body is different. Making adjustments in your exercises at this stage of the game is critical to the all-important self-confidence factor. Researchers suggest that an individual's perceived lack of skill in performing an exercise is more likely to turn him into a quitter than his lack of time.

Here are some suggestions that might make life easier for you, courtesy of Wayne Westcott, Ph.D., the YMCA's national strength-training consultant and *Men's Health* magazine advisor.

- *Tall men* have a disadvantage when it comes to doing press-type exercises. Squats, for example, put a lot of pressure on a tall man's back and knees. Do seated leg presses instead. You may want to substitute machines for free weights when doing other types of presses as well. "A good Nautilus-type machine should even things out," says Dr. Westcott.

- *Shorter men* may have more trouble with machines, since they may have to pad the seats to fit into them. Free weights may be a better bet.

- If you have *knee troubles*, avoid squats and lunges and opt for leg presses, extensions and curls instead.

- If you have *elbow or shoulder pain*, you're better off using dumbbells instead of a barbell. Tennis elbow, in particular, can cause trouble when you do military presses or triceps extensions with a bar. "Using dumbbells takes a lot of stress off the shoulders, elbows and wrists," Dr. Westcott says.

March

The Goal: Increase the intensity of your workout by setting and reaching specific targets for each exercise.

The Program: Add additional weight to each station, boosting sets to 75 percent of your maximum. Increase heart-rate target to 65 percent of maximum during aerobic exercise.

You've now been working out for about eight weeks, and you should be feeling a little stronger, a little trimmer. You've found the exercises that you're comfortable with. Now it's time to go for the gusto.

But that doesn't mean piling on all the iron you can find and straining until the folks down the block can hear you grunting. Instead, you want to increase your weight at each station until you can do no more than two sets of eight to ten repetitions of each exercise. All you need to build muscle is one or two sets, says Dr. Westcott. Anything beyond that won't make your muscles grow any better. Remember to give yourself a minute or more of rest between sets.

Once you've found the weight that will give you the maximum benefit, you have an immediate, automatic goal: to move up five to ten pounds. You'll know you've reached it when you can do more than ten repetitions on the second set. Increase the weight slightly and get working on making it to the next level.

To maximize your muscle-building ability, adopt an aerobic activity that uses the upper body as well as the lower: Rowing machines or cross-country ski machines will enhance your overall weight training, whereas running or biking build only the legs.

SPRING: A TIME FOR MELTING (FAT)

The first breezes of summer—hidden behind those 50-degree days—are in the air. And while it's too cold to be going shirtless, it is time to think about what you'll look like when you do.

And to start doing something about it.

You've built up some muscle, but now's the time to shift emphasis from overall fitness to defining those muscles. This three-month toning program is a perfect follow-up to the base work you put in during the winter.

• •

Switch to a Higher Gear

If fat is your foe, research suggests you may not have to fight this battle standing up. Studies at Tufts University in Medford, Massachusetts, measured daylong energy expenditures among men and determined that, while active men were significantly leaner, the kinds of activity they got were not necessarily traditional exercise. Such unstrenuous exertions as shifting in your chair, pacing around your office and even getting excited about a good idea add up to more calories burned, in the course of 16 waking hours, than a half-hour of sweating at the gym, explains Susan Roberts, Ph.D., chief of the Energy Metabolism Laboratory at the U.S. Department of Agriculture Human Nutrition Research Center at Tufts. "Whatever you do all day, do it vigorously," Dr. Roberts urges.

One caveat: Now that you're exercising seriously, your metabolism is increasing, and with it your appetite. Remember that no amount of exercise will burn off enough fat to compensate for deep-dish pizza binges. "Stay away from the fats," warns James Kenney, Ph.D., R.D., nutrition research specialist at the Pritikin Longevity Center in Santa Barbara, California. "If you're hungry, eat more carbohydrates like rice, pasta, fruits, potatoes and beans." Being strict about your diet at this stage of the game will help you reach your next three-month goal: to get a toned, firmer physique.

April

The Goal: To continue rapid muscle growth and avoid the dreaded exercise plateau.

The Program: Adopt a series of exercise variations to the Core Workout on page 224. Add sport-specific exercises.

You've begun an intense weight-training program, and you should be seeing gains quickly. But somewhere along the way, your gains will begin to level off. This is called the plateau, where effort expended no longer seems matched by strength gained. It's also where a lot of men become disheartened and drop out.

Monotony is the problem. "The body is going to become bored with the same program over and over," explains Darryn Willoughby, Ph.D., director of operations and research at the Center for Health and Fitness at Hood General Hospital in Granbury, Texas. "You need to vary the program. Then the body has to respond, and it can respond quite dramatically."

- Substitute a new exercise for each muscle group. (See "Alternative Exercises" in the Core Workout on page 224.) Changing just one exercise each week will keep challenging your muscles and making them grow.

- Lift less weight. A study Dr. Willoughby conducted showed that men who combined periods of high-intensity and low-intensity exercise made greater strength gains overall than those who stayed with heavy weights continuously.

- Add sport-specific exercises. While you're fiddling with your program, keep in mind that summer's coming, and with it softball games, volleyball league and an occasional weekend chasing your boss around the golf course. Choices include:

Racket sports. Seated barbell twists to strengthen oblique abdominal muscles used in all shots. (Sitting on a bench, place an unweighted barbell across your shoulders and behind your neck. Keep your head straight and slowly twist from side to side.) Exercises that strengthen the lower back will help to improve your serve.

Softball. Light shoulder exercises for throwing; wrist curls to strengthen forearms. (Sit on a bench, forearms resting on your thighs, wrists over your knees. Hold a pair of dumbbells palms up. Lower and raise the dumbbells as far as possible.)

Volleyball/basketball. Plyometric exercises such as the rim jump to put bounce into those legs. (Standing beside a wall, jump up and reach a spot about six inches higher than you can reach while standing. Do two sets of ten jumps.)

Golf. Seated barbell twists to strengthen oblique abdominal muscles; wrist curls for strong forearms.

May

The Goal: Begin toning muscle and concentrating on cutting fat.

The Program: Boost the aerobic benefit of your workout by adapting it for a circuit routine. Add additional stomach exercises to firm your gut.

● ●

Switch Blading

Studies show that running or cycling gives you a better aerobic workout than in-line skating does. But that's no reason to trade in your blades. You can easily turn up the intensity of your workout by finding a long, gradual incline and repeatedly skating up it, then resting by walking back down the hill. In-line skating uphill provides an aerobic workout you would only get at dangerously high speeds on flat ground.

Up to now, you've been working on building muscle, but with spring arriving, it's not a bad idea to place the emphasis on cutting down the amount of fat you're wearing as well as toning and shaping the muscle you have built.

The best way to do both is to make the weight lifting a bit more aerobic. This way you'll reduce the amount of fat covering your muscles, so the clear lines that define them will become apparent.

- Work in a circle. Instead of doing two back-to-back sets of each exercise, do one set at each station, then move on to the next. After you've completed one whole circuit, go back and do a second. Cut the rest between each exercise to about 30 to 45 seconds.

- Use lighter weights. David Pearson, Ph.D., of Ball State University's Human Performance Lab in Muncie, Indiana, suggests you shift to a weight you can lift 12 to 15 times to tone up the muscles.

Continue with your regular aerobic exercise (running, biking, etc.) as well, but one day a week, add an additional ten minutes to it to help build your endurance.

Finally, focus on the stomach. Beach weather is almost here, and you don't want to spend every weekend holding your breath in. To help blast the stomach, add the following stomach exercises to the Core Workout from page 224: Two sets of incline, bent-knee crunches, followed by two sets of seated crunches and two sets of bent-knee leg raises.

June

The Goal: Boost your aerobic endurance, increasing the difficulty and duration of your aerobic workout.

The Program: Cut back to doing only the Core Workout routine twice a week, 12 repetitions on each circuit with less rest. The third day of exercise should go to a continuous aerobic activity.

For all intents and purposes, summer is here. You're already spending time by the pool, and it's getting harder and harder to force yourself indoors to work out. That's why it's time to channel some energy into outdoor activities: running, cycling, power walking, hiking, even rowing if you have access to a boat.

In addition, increase the benefits you're getting from stomach exercises by placing a ten-pound weight plate across your chest for added resistance.

SUMMER: TURNING UP THE HEAT

It's warm, it's sunny, and the last place you want to be is inside a hot, sweaty gym. The good news is you're not going to have to confine yourself to the weight room in order to maintain all the muscle you've built. "Studies have shown that you can maintain the strength you've gained with one workout a week," says Dr. Westcott. "Once you've gotten a muscle to a level, it doesn't take a lot of stimulus to keep it there."

But you must make that once-a-week trip. "If you drop out of a weight program altogether, in just three months you'll lose up to 70 percent of what you gained," says James Graves, Ph.D., chairman of the Health and Physical Education Program at Syracuse University in New York.

To keep your aerobic workout interesting, mix things up. Bike one day. Go kayaking the next. Run, walk, whatever. Just be sure to get out there.

July

The Goal: Try to increase aerobic activity by 10 percent a week.

The Program: Cut your weight workout to once a week, adding an additional day of pure aerobic exercise.

One day a week, repeat the Core Workout on page 224, including warm-up and cooldown.

Then, for your other *two days*, get outside for a continuous aerobic activity. Start slowly and shoot for time (40 minutes), not distance or speed. The point is to exercise consistently, not to run yourself into the ground. "Like muscle, endurance takes time to build," says Ken Sparks, Ph.D., an exercise physiologist at Cleveland State University and world-class masters runner. "If you can only do 20 minutes the first week, try to increase by 10 percent the next week and so on."

August

The Goal: Increase aerobic benefits without increasing the amount of time spent. Avoid aerobic plateau.

The Program: Integrate interval-training techniques into one session of aerobic exercise per week.

Continuous aerobic exercise will only take you so far, says Dr. Sparks. "Interval training will give you substantially more speed and power." One day a week, warm up with five minutes of aerobic exercise, say, jogging, then lift the pace sharply, such as by sprinting for 30 seconds. The same effect can be had with a bicycle, jump rope, rower, and so on, just as long as it leaves you panting. After 30 seconds, slow down for two minutes or until your breathing levels off a bit. Repeat the cycle two or three times. Work up to six repetitions. Be sure to cool down with easy exercise to facilitate muscle recovery for the next workout.

AUTUMN: DON'T QUIT NOW

At this point, you have a good base—now build on it. A little more endurance, a little more power—with a little extra work here and there, your flexibility, strength and stamina will improve by significant increments.

September

The Goal: Discover how far your aerobic training has taken you. Continue to push the envelope.

The Program: Target one aerobic session per week as an endurance test.

Weight lifting is going to stay the same. But switch one day's aerobic workout to the weekend, making it longer. Your goal is to run or bike or row or swim a little bit farther each week. Add ten minutes to your aerobic activity this month.

On your other two exercise days, boost your intervals by making them more frequent and longer-lasting. For example, sprint for 30 seconds and jog for only 30 seconds (instead of the full two minutes as in the August plan). Increase the sprinting portion by 10 seconds per session until it's one full minute.

With the weather turning colder, you can begin to ease back into the gym and start concentrating on building muscle. Since you maintained a once-a-week weight routine throughout the summer, jumping back in to an intense weight-lifting schedule shouldn't be too hard. You also want to strengthen your legs for winter, especially if you're a skier.

October

The Goal: To build muscle with weights and avoid burnout from aerobic activity. Strengthen legs and improve flexibility.

The Program: Return to the Core Workout two days a week. Trail running one day a week.

It's still nice outside, but winter is around the bend. Even if you don't ski, this is a good time to improve your leg strength and flexibility.

- *Trail running.* In addition to putting you right in the midst of the autumn foliage, running trails will also build muscle and help improve your balance. "Trail running on hilly terrain works more of the hip flexors, the arms and the back than running on the flat," says David Martin, Ph.D., an exercise physiologist at Georgia State University in Atlanta. Running at the shallow end of an indoor pool is a great alternative for those who live in urban or flat areas.

- *Mountain biking.* If you're a cyclist, mountain biking is trail running's two-wheeled cousin.

November

The Goal: Assess individual weaknesses and attack muscles that were neglected during the summer.

The Program: Return to Core Workout three days a week. Put extra weight-training emphasis on specific muscles that need improvement.

This is the month to target muscles that got a free ride during your summer aerobic workouts. For example, if you cy-

• •

Flat Wrong

Flat feet used to be a soldier's ticket out of the service, because it was thought that they made him injury prone. A study of 246 male army recruits shows that flat-footed people are less prone to injury from exercising than are people with higher arches. Recruits with the highest arches had a six-times-greater injury risk than their flat-footed chums.

cled during the summer, you should have great quadriceps but are likely to have weak hamstrings. If you ran, you have the opposite condition. If you played tennis, focus on the shoulder or hip muscles of the nondominant side.

Up the intensity. One day a week, enhance your weight-training gains with reverse pyramid sets. To do this, complete two sets of an exercise with a weight you can lift eight to ten times. But at the end of the second set, when you can no longer generate the force to lift that weight again, immediately shift to a lower weight that you can lift and continue with the exercise until you are fully fatigued. Some believe that this technique stimulates the muscles to grow even more.

December

The Goal: Get through the month without missing a workout.

The Program: Replace one day's weight training with a dumbbell workout.

If there's one month that just demands that you fall off your training schedule, it's December. Not only will there be shopping, visiting relatives, office parties and the like, but your work schedule is likely to be more hectic as you try to cram a month's worth of business in before the 25th.

The trick? Drop out in advance. Buy yourself an early Christmas present: a set of adjustable dumbbells. Whenever you can't get to the gym, set aside an hour at night or the next morning to put yourself through the paces. "You can use the same dumbbell to do almost an infinite variety of exercises," says Dr. Graves. One caveat: If you generally work with exercise machines instead of free weights, use a slightly lower weight when you start with the dumbbells. Learning to balance them can take some practice, says Dr. Graves, and you don't want to show up at the office party without your front teeth.

There you have it. Fifty-two weeks of fitness guaranteed to get you in shape and keep you there. So next New Year's Day, you'll look in the mirror and won't be flabbergasted by the flab. The house, however, will probably still be a mess.

—Dave Kuehls

Part 9

TAKING CARE
OF BUSINESS

How to Impress the Boss

*Think that big guy they call your boss doesn't need
his share of mercy and kindness? Think again. Here
are eight ways to make nice when it counts.*

• • • • • • • • • • • • • • • • • •

HOW DO YOU TELL SOMEONE you love them? Particularly when mere words will not suffice?

For a family member, the task is relatively simple. Material objects of varying economic heft and weft are both called for and expected. These may include but not be limited to cameras, Sega Game Gear (the particular choice of the local gods of greed around here), in-line skates, lingerie (for my wife) and an item of computer hardware that costs a real lot for the whole family (although I'll probably get the most use out of it). That, as I said, is the easy stuff. All it requires is funding.

Establishing a statement of affection without money is another thing altogether. And yet that's the task that for the most part faces you in business, creating an aura of profound regard on occasions for the benevolent masters of the mountain horde, good folks, really, who under no circumstances would you ever want to alienate—especially at their most emotionally vulnerable points of the year (like right before you're about to receive your annual review). At times like these, you want them to know that you consider them part of your extended family.

So how is one to express that without money? Since overt sucking up seems, sadly, to have fallen out of favor, what's required is a way to give your boss some very special treatment. What you're looking for are deep, existential quality-of-life improvements, essential spiritual niceties he may be too shy or lacking in insight to ask you for. Read on for eight ways to show him just how much you really and truly do love him and recognize his enormous needs as a human being.

● ●

Another Good Reason to Hate Your Boss

More evidence that high-pressure deadlines at work can trigger heart-daunting stress: Experimenters in London monitored the physical reactions of 40 middle-age men who were given identical problem-solving tasks. Blood pressure and heart rate jumped significantly higher in the men who had to perform at a rate set by the experimenters, compared with those who worked at their own pace. These classic signs of stress were particularly severe in the men who reported feeling lots of strain in their real-world jobs. The obvious lesson in all this? Finding ways to gain more control over tasks at work and pacing yourself so you don't feel so rushed can keep stress in check.

First thing in the day, try to implement a morning buzz-by. Sure, the manager in question could call you in any time and requisition some affection or, lacking that, activity. But when was the last time you simply dropped by at 8:47 A.M. and stood about with a cup of coffee in your hand, oozing gossip and goodwill before trundling off on your merry way? It's amazing how a morning moment of humanity can soften the buffer between the first anxieties of the early hours and the rolling hamster wheel of the rest of the day. Simply lean on your man's (or woman's) door quietly until he or she notices you. A simple "How's it goin'" or "Whazzup?" will then set things off on the right path.

LEND HIM YOUR EAR

By 9:07 A.M., if things are going well, it'll be time to offer your second gift—a human ear. If you sit there, he will talk. For a while he will disgorge a welter of business chat, pearls of strategic wisdom or, lacking that, orders. After that, he'll start getting anxious. As a group, bosses tend to suffer from the belief that they are boring to other people when the subject is not strictly business. Nonsense, right? Give him that ear and he'll take your whole head. That's all right. You weren't doing anything more important with it anyway, were you?

By 10, you will probably be out of his office and up to doing whatever it is you do. Do it quickly, because by 10:50 it'll be time to give him gift number three—freedom from the responsibility to be human. There's nothing more exhausting to a boss than an employee who, just because he was your friend at 8:00 A.M., thinks he's still your friend at 9:15. So when your boss walks by you on the way to a meeting two hours after your toasty morning chat and doesn't say hello or anything, let him off the hook. Don't fester. His status relieves him of the duty to build on existing personal relationships like normal people in normal settings, and any guilt you make him feel, any attitude you strike that questions his right to be curt, perfunctory or bizarre is a drain on his powerpack. Give the gift of emotional deniability. He'll be glad you did.

And he'll be back. Right before lunch, remembering that you have more on the ball than he sometimes gives you credit for, he'll be asking you to take one of his wasteful, brain-dead projects onto your shoulders. Consider that gift number four. You may have to do some work to get at it, though. Don't worry. During the course of any conversation, a boss will molt problems and unresolved desires and issues much in the same way a junkyard dog walks about in a cloud of fleas. Listen hard, and, when the time seems opportune, take a tough one. For example:

For example, a couple of months ago, my pal Nagle was grabbing a cup of coffee (standing up) in the nook opposite the executive suite. His boss, Mr. Brewster, walked out with a harried expression.

"Coffee?" said Nagle.

"Sure," said Brewster.

"Bad morning?" said Nagle.

"Nah," said Brewster. "I just hate my ceiling."

"Your . . . ceiling?" said Nagle.

"It's brown," said Brewster. "Makes the whole room feel cramped and . . . claustrophobic."

Over the weekend, Nagle had the Office Services people paint Brewster's ceiling white. On Monday, there it was. He called Nagle in immediately. "Somebody's done something to my office, Fred," he said to Nagle suspiciously. "But I can't put my finger on it."

Nagle told him. Brewster slammed him on the back for a couple of hours and hasn't really stopped doing so ever since. "I like Nagle," he told me just last week. "The guy is a risk-taker and a strategic thinker."

I had to agree.

At lunchtime, you'll go downstairs to "grab a sandwich," which in my company means sitting down for about 90 minutes over some seriously excellent veal. This gives you a chance to exercise your next gift option: picking up the check. Why, you may ask, when the fellow across the radicchio makes at least five times what you do and can sign for up to a million dollars without reaching the limits of his authority? Because, no matter how big he is, his expense report must go to someone. You give your form to him. He gives his to the Central Politburo in Moscow. Who's going to be more likely to see that $34.27 as a thoroughly righteous business expense?

THE GIFT OF SILENCE

Back from lunch, as you putter about in the valley of fatigue between 2:00 and 3:30, you can give the gift of silence. There's a host of horrible stuff he's delegated to you over the course of the last few months. Several of the most detestable projects he hasn't even asked about in . . . how long has it been? Long enough. Know why? Because he doesn't want to hear about it. That problem, for instance, with the industry luncheon table that he committed $2,500 to, only to find out that the chairman had turned down the same request for funds just the day before with the words "This has got to be the most idiotic idea of a luncheon I've ever come across."

After that, your boss thrust the already-signed contract for his table in your face and said, "Get out of this." Which you did, in one of the most adroit moves you've ever accomplished, moving the obligation over to one of your out-of-town subsidiaries who actually had a good reason to be there. What a coup! So why does he glaze over when you want to crow about it? Because he's not proud of it, and no glory at all redounds to him, that's why! When he wants to hear about stuff, tell him. That's the bottom line.

Unless the shark he's trying to ignore is about to come up from the depths and bite him in the executive function. In

● ●

Fight That Twitch

Can't sell that time share in Florida? Maybe you have an annoying little habit that's getting in the way. Psychology researchers at Texas Christian University in Fort Worth have determined that people who make weird gestures seem insincere. In a study, college students were shown videotapes of people talking. Some of the speakers had been instructed to raise a shoulder to an ear, lift an arm to the ceiling or show some other bizarre behavior. It turned out that the students were more likely to judge that the speaker was lying if he acted strangely.

that case, give him the gift that keeps on giving: a human shield. That's you, Bud. At some point or another down the road, this may mean taking a bullet for him but not now. Not today. Today we're going to make his life better by taking the conference call on corporate giving so he doesn't have to do it. He's going to the jewelry store to buy his wife a necklace for their anniversary instead. Isn't that nice?

The day is almost done. Yet there are so many presents left unpresented! Given the lateness of the hour and the impossibility of the task, it doesn't look like you're going to be able to give him the head of Dickie Stritch on a sharp stick, as he asked you to do not long ago. No, it looks like the shareholder's advocate and general geek will live another year to harass and torment the corporation at the annual stockholder's meeting. Nor will you be able to give him the liver of Biff Krentz, your CEO, on a platter, for all the projects he's dinged in the past two years. The best you'll be able to offer is the unpleasant information that the marketing plan he's been working on is in serious trouble with Weaver, Krentz and Boskin, the three guys who supersede him in the organizational chart. You heard about this from Krentz himself, who seems to like you a lot and even trust you some.

Be that as it may. This tidbit of rancid news is something your guy should know, definitely. So you give it to him. And spend a half-hour or so with the poor, beleaguered dude as you both stand in the corridor with your topcoats on, scheming, planning, spinning the big monster of tomorrow until it looks almost human.

You're a good man, you know that?

Maybe that's the best gift of all.

—Gil Schwartz

Don't Get Burned

Your job may go up in smoke. A prominent career counselor offers the next best thing to a "fired" insurance policy.

• • • • • • • • • • • • • • • • • • •

MEN DON'T LIKE TO THINK about getting fired or laid off. But the fact is, the ax does fall occasionally, often through downsizing, restructuring, i.e., through no fault of one's own. That's why it's essential to be prepared for the worst even when your job seems perfectly secure. We talked to Harvey Mackay, best-selling author of *Sharkproof: Get the Job You Want, Keep the Job You Love . . . in Today's Frenzied Job Market*, about the importance of being ready for any eventuality.

What would you say is the most important principle of job survival?

Dig your well before you're thirsty. In other words, be ready to be fired. When you get up in the morning, ask yourself, "What would I do and where would I go if I got terminated today? What can I do *now* to make the transition easier?" Often, the steps you take will make it less likely that you'll be let go in the first place.

Specifically, what are some of those steps?

Establish contacts at every meeting you go to, every airplane you ride on, every conference, every cocktail party. Then make sure to keep in touch with those people. You'll need them someday, and they'll need you.

Does education fit into your plan?

Realize that you don't go to school once anymore. You go for your entire career. And I'm not talking only about formal classes. The person who wants to hang on to his job has to practice his skills and continually broaden them. Get familiar with every aspect of your industry and acquire as much general knowledge outside your field as possible. If you don't know anything about accounting, go to night school and take a course. If you're not a strong public speaker, join Toastmasters International. Being a generalist makes you more valuable as an employee, and more marketable as a jobseeker. There's no way in the 1990s that you can just stand still.

How do you keep a career on track through the rough spots?

There's no substitute for having a mentor who'll give you good advice. Every successful person in all fields of endeavor, whether he's a Pavarotti or a Ping-Pong player, became successful because others helped him along the way.

If you're not lucky enough to have a mentor, the next best thing to do is study successful people. Find the common threads and apply whatever is practical to you.

Finally, have goals. A goal is a dream with a deadline. Measurable, identifiable, containable, specific—and in writing.

—*Richard Laliberte*

Business Travel Cheap-'n'-Easy

Flying for business doesn't have to be expensive. If you're smart, you can get more comfort and less hassle for fewer dollars.

● ● ● ● ● ● ● ● ● ● ● ● ● ● ● ● ● ● ●

NO MATTER WHAT THE NEWSWEEKLY trend-spotters tell us about the brave new info-world—e-mail, TV over the phone lines, home shopping, virtual sex—at some point in the not-too-distant future, we will have to raise those millions of sluggish bodies from the pale reality of our satellite-fed living rooms and move them around the Earth. Physically. Your body and my body. Most especially my body, but I'll get to that later. I am talking about the fact that some information about the world is actually unavailable via your cable system. I am talking about the fact that in the not-too-distant future, inevitably, you and I are going to have to travel. How do we travel, or more precisely, how do we travel best? Alexander the Great didn't bother with luggage; he simply pillaged his way across what then became his empire, sort of picking up luggage (gilt cauldrons, art, extra tents, elephants, concubines) as he went along. Of course, he had the advantage of traveling with hordes of fanatically loyal, heavily armed soldiers to do his slightest bidding, which simplified the road for him in a way that is no longer possible for us.

A bridge of land to that island redoubt? Sixty of those vestal virgins? No problem, Your Excellency!

Travel is, in fact, tough. I have been traveling to get my work done, without an attendant army of fanatically loyal soldiers, for 17 years, and I'd like to share some of this hard-won knowledge with you. The idea these days is not to spend three or four years conquering the countries you visit but to get there and leave quickly once your business or vacationing is done. The modern art of travel is about the manipulation of time.

• •

Learning to Love Home Work

If "working at home" brings to mind the solitary seamstress or the lonely writer, consider this: A nine-state survey found that 7 percent of workers had home-based jobs. Contrary to expectations, the majority (55 percent) of workers in the study were men. Home-based workers put in about as many hours as outside workers and make less money, the survey found. But they're a lot happier than people who work in an office or a factory.

"It's a lifestyle choice," says researcher Barbara Rowe, Ph.D., associate professor of consumer sciences and retailing at Purdue University in West Lafayette, Indiana. "They feel very much in control of when they work, how they work and how much. If they want to program software in the basement in the middle of the night, stark naked, they can do it."

Unfortunately, this requires the use of aircraft, credit cards, languages other than your own, telephones, hotels and, more often than not, your health in the form of your digestive system and your internal clock. It's not my job to make everybody paranoid, but we must think of a trip as one machine with many highly calibrated tolerances, a sort of finely spun Ferrari that is liable to take you where you want to go in great style and very quickly—but just as liable to blow up in your face.

Essentially, given the modern world's time constraints and the distances involved, if you want to travel today you have no choice but to fly. Do you understand what it means to have no choice? It means that the airline companies can do with you what they will. No matter how small and funereal the dessicated, shrink-wrapped sandwich, no matter how surly and obtuse the help, no matter how closely the pain in your cramped legs resembles the bends, you will still fly because flying is the only way to go.

THE GOOD OLD DAYS

Ironically, before the age of air travel, the world was not much *less* but rather much *more* one place. Time ran in one direction and at one speed. You took time to take a trip. This adds up to one very simple but very important fact: Without jets, there is no jet lag.

Lag, or the sudden displacement of the human body by means of a jet into another part of the world with a significant time difference, is arguably the main travel difficulty we face, or more accurately, it is one of the most constant difficulties. You can depend on jet lag in the way that you depend on your body's internal clock. In fact, lag happens precisely because you have an internal clock.

Lag is also the author of our problems with airplanes in general—space, food, noise level, proximity to the toilet and the enormous Middle Eastern gentleman who, simply as a result of his unavoidable size, absorbs your armrest under the folds of his robes. None of these minor discomforts would matter if we were talking about a short hop. But as the ill-fitting shoe results in blisters if worn long enough, minor discomforts grow to major irritations in proportion to the length of the trip. And not only must you endure them, when they've been removed you must pay for the whole trip in the form of the disorienting sort of time/space hangover we call jet lag.

Some people engage in yoga to fight it off; others turn themselves into urine factories, consuming gallons of designer water to rehydrate themselves; others try to drink themselves into an alcoholic haze, presumably so that they feel so bad from a traditional hangover that they don't notice the more fundamental dislocation of the lag. Others simply succumb. I have tried all of the above. None of them work because none of them address the fundamental chemical problem.

RESET YOUR INNER CLOCK

The body's internal clock lies in the brain. The "clock," located in the hypothalamus, is actually a bundle of nerve receptors called the suprachiasmatic nuclei or scn. The scn are regulated by a hormone called melatonin, which is generated in the pineal gland. This substance, manufactured at night (when the clock perceives it is dark), essentially tells the appropriate receptors (the clock itself) how your day is going to progress, i.e., when to turn the motor of your body on, so to speak, how many hours you'll be needing to keep it running and when to get tired and go to sleep. Regardless of what you have planned. Lag is simply the problem that this clock, with the help of a jet, no longer matches the run of the day in which the body finds itself.

The nation's premier researcher in this arena is Al Lewy, M.D., Ph.D., professor of psychiatry at Oregon Health Sciences University in Portland. He and his colleagues are in the process of developing a synthetic melatonin for long-distance travelers and people with sleep disorders. "Basically, we know where the clock is and how melatonin binds in the brain," he says. "If you take melatonin in the morning, it makes you think it is still dark out, and you'll shift your body clock later (the strategy for traveling west). If you take it later in the day, it will make you think that it's getting dark before it does, and you'll shift your clock earlier (for traveling east)."

Brilliant! There's just one problem. Synthetic melatonin is still in the approval stages and will take up to four years to get to the shelves. There is, however, something we can do now, according to Dr. Lewy. Our internal clocks are sensitive not simply to darkness (when melatonin is produced) but also to sunlight. The strategy, therefore, pending the approval of melatonin, is to drive your clock forward or back by exposing yourself to sunlight at given times of day, thus triggering the clock to pull itself forward or push itself back. Dr. Lewy says, "If you're traveling six time zones or fewer to the east, you should try to catch the first few hours of daylight to pull your clock to the beginning of the day; if you're traveling to the west, you should catch the light in the late afternoon. More than six time zones to the east, avoid the A.M. light. More than six time zones west, avoid outdoor light in the late afternoon."

I haven't yet had the pleasure of engaging in this human photosynthesis, but I'm tickled about trying.

PLANE FACTS

We must deal with certainly the ugliest circumstance of our inquiry, namely, the method of conveyance. I'm going to be talking about planes here, but first a few ground rules. As stated, I'm not going to deal with short hops. They don't matter, and what's more, I'm angry at short hops, because I cannot stand the idea that some people are getting away with less discomfort than me. My problem is that I only take long hops. For two years I've been working between New York and Berlin, averaging four to six trips of a month or longer per year. In fact, you could call me a commuter—it's just my tough luck that I've drawn a commute of 6,908 miles, round trip, as my frequent-flyer newsletters relentlessly inform me.

I want to introduce you to a new word: "equipment," as in what sort of equipment we flyin'? This is a paramount question for you to be asking. This question—and I mean exactly this question and no other—telegraphs the subtextual message that the traveler using the word has been around the block. It is a question that may or may not get you better service and/or a better seat, but at least it'll open the discussion so that you get the chance.

In order to use that chance, you have to get to know the equipment itself. I've been flying the new Airbus A-300 a lot to Berlin. Occasionally, I'll luck out and get the really roomy Boeing 747—or the more compact L-1011—but more often than not it's the Airbus, which in my view richly deserves its name.

It's a European-manufactured piece of equipment, and, like the houses in Amsterdam or the toilets in Paris, they've designed every available square centimeter of space out of that plane. It is tight, brand-new and very efficient, but efficiency in aircraft design is, for the passengers anyway, a double-edge sword. There used to be corners in the old 747s, a couple of square feet of turning room near the galleys, and standing space next to the really broad emergency exits. You could move around in those planes. They were beamy as nineteenth-century schooners. But they were less efficient.

The comforting thing about those planes—the comforting thing about any good plane—is that you have a reassuring sense that there's somewhere else in the vessel that you can go besides your seat. This doesn't have to be an actual place so much as an illusion of place. It's obviously not so critical a point in first or business class, but it is a dire situation in economy. Whether it's the exigencies of carry-on baggage—which we'll get to in a moment—or simply the crying need after six hours or so on board to stretch one's legs, you need a seat with a view.

STARE AT THE WALL

In the 747s, the best seats in economy were obviously bulkhead, or aisle seats in the emergency-exit rows, but I'd like to remind people who live by bulkhead seats that what they are doing for six to seven hours at a stretch is basically staring at a wall.

In the aptly named Airbus, the emergency-exit rows are no great shakes—with their new, cruelly efficient design, those delicious few extra centimeters of space have been cut back, so they feel an awful lot like all the other rows.

The strategy on the Airbus? Ask for the aisle seats in rows 20 or 21, which are the break between business and economy. Try not to get the seats in the middle section, because that is most likely to be the place (in a plane configured two-four-two) in which they've clustered those heartbreakingly cute new parents with children. This means that you, as their neighbor, are going to spend the next seven hours fielding the soppy napkins, buttered rolls and glasses of fruit juice that will be flung about your seat while you inspect, at close range, parts of other people's anatomy that, frankly, you get to see enough of at home.

My buddy and travel agent, the intrepid Stanley Rhodes of Linden Travel in New York City, who flies a hundred thousand miles a year, on average, advises the following: If you're traveling with somebody you care about, get your agent to "block" a row, that is, put one of you at one end of a row and the other at the other end. This works best when the section is configured for three seats only. The idea here is that very few people want a seat in the middle of a row, and if the flight is not crowded, you have a row to yourselves. If the flight is crowded, you have either the aisle or the window to trade in order to sit next to your loved one.

THE WORST SEAT

There are several other Rhodesian tips: The worst seat on any plane—and statistically one of the safest in a crash, by the way—is in the last row. Why? Because the rear bulkhead prevents those seats from reclining. On the Airbus, as on most other aircraft, the last few rows (rows 33 to 38) are where the plane narrows, and so there are almost always fewer people back this way, but this is also the place where it takes much, much longer to get off the damn plane. I mean, you could be ordering a meal in a restaurant in town while these guys are back there still waiting to disembark and watching their beards grow in.

Which brings me to another touchy transcontinental health topic: smoking. Although smoking has been banned on domestic flights, the back rows of most long flights are devoted to people who need to smoke even in confined spaces. If you've spent any time in eastern or central Europe, you'll understand when I say that in most of those countries, tobacco is considered a vegetable. In these places, people think you are a

THE BEST SEATS IN THE HOUSE

Not all airplane seats are created equal. Here are a few tips on getting the greatest amount of elbowroom.

Roomiest Aircraft: 767s and MD-80s

Most Cramped Aircraft: 757s and 737s, which also have the fewest restrooms per capita.

Roomiest Airline: TWA, which increased the space between rows of seats on its airplanes from 31 to 36 inches.

Safest Seats: Anywhere in back. Studies have shown the back third of an aircraft is up to 34 percent safer than the front. Exception: the 727-100. It lacks rear side exits, and its rear airstair exit may be unusable in a gear-up landing, because it is located underneath the airplane.

Most Comfortable Seats: Exit rows because they help you avoid kids (federal regulations prohibit children in these rows), and aisle seats in the center section because the seats next to them are the last to be filled.

little strange, weak, unserious—at best, of a light constitution—if you do not smoke. What does this mean? It means that the planes en route to and from such romantic destinations as Prague or Moscow are going to be filled with smoke. It means that in a very real sense there is no such thing as a nonsmoking section. It means: Turn your air on and get used to it, or take the boat to Leningrad.

CARRY ON

The basic notion is that you must be able to expand on an airplane, preferably in all directions but at least in two: in baggage and in legroom. For this reason I must order you to take one, and only one, carry-on bag. And you must, you absolutely must, get an aisle seat. But sometimes even these things aren't enough.

I'm six-foot-two, and I like to work on planes. I find it restful and somehow wonderful that I'm out of reach of a phone. This requires space, often more space than is offered in a simple economy seat. So I grab a mountain of newspapers, make sure that I have extra batteries for the Walkman and the laptop, and whack away. Here's the rather ugly but self-preservative point: Jamming a couple of hundred people into a metal tube for six or seven (or eight or ten) hours at a stretch is an aggressive thing for airline companies to do. They'd like us to think that they're offering us adventure and friendly skies, but they do it to make a profit, and so they jam as many of us as closely together as possible. That is what an airline actually does, as opposed to what it appears to do. It's therefore useful to violate the social contract just enough so that the employees regard you with respect and your fellow passengers leave you alone. There's nothing like a sleek, humming little laptop, a Walkman and a pair of wraparound shades—all on at the same time—to telegraph that ominous professional traveler's don't-mess-with-me! message.

Perhaps all that travel boils down to is a simple little list of self-preservative rules: (1) Be unfriendly, because you can always be friendly later. (2) Suck out of your opponents, your airline, and your fellow man every morsel of advantage that you can. And (3) have a wonderful, wonderful time.

—*Guy Martin*

Wing Tips

Fifty-six timesaving, comfort-raising, cost-cutting secrets from men who depend on the airplane for their livelihood.

• • • • • • • • • • • • • • • • • • •

HAVE YOU NOTICED THAT somewhere between your first boyhood dream of exploring the Amazon jungle and your last business trip to Des Moines, travel has ceased to be an adventure of the spirit and has grown to be a big pain in the seat? Maybe it was the umpteenth overdue, overbooked flight that did it. Perhaps it was one too many microwaved airplane chicken breasts. Whatever the cause, the thrill is gone, replaced by weary resignation.

Unless you know the ropes. There are ways to ease the discomfort of long hours crammed in a flying sardine can, ways to cut down on wasted time getting to and from the airport—ways to make the whole process smooth as silk. We asked dozens of public figures, men who depend for their livelihood on the airplane, for their most valuable travel tips. Here's what they had to say.

MAKING RESERVATIONS

Alan Rachins, *actor, L.A. Law:* Never let them give you the bulkhead seat. That's the one in front of the cabin that doesn't have another seat in front of it and, therefore, doesn't have anywhere for you to store your carry-on baggage.

Paul Prudhomme, *chef:* Always request the same seat or position, like the "A" seat in the last row of first class. Sitting in the same spot makes it easier to sleep, because it becomes almost familiar, like going to sleep in your own bed.

John Paul Jones Dejoria, *CEO, Paul Mitchell Salon Haircare:* Tell your travel agent you want to choose between a $100 hotel, a $150 hotel and a $200 hotel, and ask her to give you the address of each. If you decide to stay at the $150 hotel and then find it doesn't meet your standards, you still have the name and address of the $200 hotel. Or, if you find you're running a little short on funds, you also have the name and address of the $100 hotel.

Riddick Bowe, *former world heavyweight boxing champion:* There are a lot of really nice hotels out there, but the things that are important to me are the service and the people who are providing it. I'm just as happy at a nice budget motel as I am at a Ritz-Carlton, as long as the people who work there are pleasant, mature and professional.

Robin Cook, *author,* Coma *and* Blindsight: If you want a great vacation, go to the Hotel Danieli in Venice, Italy, and stay in Room 70—but stay only about three nights.

ON-TIME RECORDS

Airline	Chance Your Plane Will Arrive within 15 Minutes of Schedule
1. Southwest	92.1%
2. America West	88.9%
3. Northwest	86.1%
4. Alaska	84.6%
5. TWA	82.1%
6. American	82.1%
7. United	81.3%
8. USAir	79.6%
9. Delta	79.1%
10. Continental	79.0%

PACKING

Kent Mercker, *pitcher, Atlanta Braves professional baseball team*: Carry a little steam iron with you—they're outstanding. And if you don't have one of those, put the clothes that need ironing in the bathroom and crank the hot water on the shower for about 15 minutes. Just don't hang your clothes on a wire hanger when you do this—the hanger will rust and leave lines on your clothes.

Lew Schneider, *actor,* Down the Shore: Pack half the number of pants you think you need and twice the amount of underwear.

Dave Barry, *syndicated columnist:* Always tighten the cap on the shampoo bottle before you put it in your suitcase. Otherwise—trust me here—it's going to leak all over everything, including your toothbrush, and when you brush your teeth you'll be foaming at the mouth as though you've been bitten by a dog infected with herbal-scented rabies.

Victor Kiam, *CEO, Remington Products:* I always travel

as if I were just going away for a few nights—you can always get your clothes cleaned by the hotel's laundry service. The only exception to that are socks. I carry one pair for every day I'm on the road. That's because when you send your clothes to the hotel laundry service, they clean them in extraordinarily hot water, and that just takes all the stretch out of them.

David Brenner, *comedian:* About six weeks before a vacation starts, I start worrying about what clothes to take. I begin putting outfits and incidentals in a closet I call my trip closet. I always overdo it. In one afternoon, in one Banana Republic store, I purchased everything anyone would need on any trip anywhere at any time of the year. Every shirt went with every pair of pants, both of which were matched with the socks, with every rain jacket and with every belt and tie.

IN AND OUT OF THE AIRPORT

Arthur C. Clarke, *author,* 2001: A Space Odyssey: I discovered, after being afflicted by postpolio syndrome, that a wheelchair makes even Heathrow painless. Of course, if everyone knew this, the result would be chaos, but I couldn't care less. I won't be there, as I plan to travel no more.

Henry Winkler, *director:* In addition to a name tag, I tie pieces of green and red ribbon around the handles of my suitcases, so I can find them immediately.

Robert Ludlum, *author,* The Scorpio Illusion: No matter where you go, take several hundred dollars of that country's currency with you when you leave the United States. It makes things much easier when you arrive not to have to rush to a money exchange before catching a taxi out of the airport or before heading to your hotel.

Robin Leach, *rich-people watcher:* Some car rental companies will deliver a car to your hotel at no extra charge, so see if you can have a limousine service take you to your hotel and get your rental car there. You don't have to worry about reading maps late at night or getting lost on dark roads, you'll get a good night's sleep and your car will be there waiting for you when you wake up in the morning.

Hugh Downs, *journalist,* 20/20: Don't skimp on car rentals. You can get a super bargain on a rental car, but then you get a less dependable car.

Joe Bob Briggs, *author,* Iron Joe Bob: When I need to rent a car, I use that Hertz "King of Sheba" executive service. I don't remember the name of it, but it's the deal where they have a car running with the keys in it, a mechanic stowed in the trunk and a bikini-clad maiden in the passenger seat ready to serve me a cold drink.

THE FLYING PART

Alan Dershowitz, *attorney and author:* The key to relaxation while flying is to take control of the environment on an airplane. I bring my own music, my own food and my own reading material. Before the flight takes off, I tell the flight attendants, politely, to please fill my cup with herbal tea periodically, and that otherwise, I don't want to be disturbed. I can make a cross-country trip and be prepared to argue a case or make a speech right off the plane.

Joseph Wambaugh, *author,* Fugitive Nights: I used to have a real fear of flying . . . coach. Once I started writing books and my publisher started flying me first class, I discovered that I wasn't really afraid of flying; I just had claustrophobia. Once I realized that, climbing on an airplane has never bothered me as much.

Jerry Seinfeld, *comedian:* I really like not dealing with people. When I'm on a plane, I always make sure to do everything the stewardess wants me to do before it needs to be done, just so she doesn't have to come over and say anything.

Robert Ludlum: Take off your shoes. A lot of people say, "Don't take off your shoes—your feet will swell," but I say, "Fine, let them—I'll walk off the plane in those little airline slippers if I have to."

Ritch Shydner, *comedian:* Get some exercise. Do some

• •

Take Your Honey for a Drink

If you've had too many drinks during a night on the town, eat some honey on crackers or toast when you get home. It will help ward off a hangover's headache and queasy stomach, according to the National Headache Foundation. Honey is loaded with fructose, which helps metabolize alcohol in your bloodstream.

stretching and walk around the aisle a bit. You may look like an idiot, but if you sit there in your seat for the entire five hours, you'll feel like a cow on the way to the slaughterhouse.

Robin Cook: Since flying often dehydrates you, I always make it a point to avoid alcohol. I take bananas with me when I fly, because one of the first things you start to lose when you dehydrate is potassium, and bananas have lots of potassium in them. I drink a lot of orange and tomato juice, and I never drink any coffee when I'm flying because that dehydrates you, too.

Ice-T, *musician:* Make sure you have clean socks on when you fly, so if you take off your shoes to get comfortable, you won't funk out the whole plane with the smell.

Pete Wilson, *governor of California:* One of my rules of thumb is to do work. There's no way I'll ever get comfortable or sleep well on a cramped airplane, so if I can't enjoy it, I might as well use it, and I'll have more time to undo my tie and enjoy myself at home.

Branford Marsalis, *musical director,* The Tonight Show: Take a CD player and some Sony MDR-V6 headphones with you when you fly. They have great bass resonance and block in all the music so you don't have to turn it up as loud, and the noise from the outside doesn't get in. Babies crying—not a problem. People talking—not a problem. You're in your own little world.

Orel Hershiser, *pitcher, Los Angeles Dodgers professional baseball team:* Ten to 15 minutes before landing, head off to the men's room to freshen up. I put on a little cologne and brush my teeth, and I wear a hair gel that can be reactivated with a little water. If my hair gets messed up when I fall asleep, I can just wet it and get it back in shape.

TRAVELING WITH CHILDREN

Jerry Mathers, *"The Beav":* Don't make the mistake of thinking that if you take your children with you on the red-eye to save a little money, they're going to sleep all the way and be bright-eyed and cheery in the morning. We tried it, and they were little terrors when we got there, because they lost an entire night's sleep.

TRAVELERS' WORK TOOLS

Peter Norton, *inventor, Norton Utilities software:* Don't travel with a high-powered laptop. Take the smallest thing that will do the job for you. For me, that's a Gateway Handbook, a notebook PC.

Peter Arnett, *correspondent, CNN:* When it comes to working on the road, I prefer a portable Canon Typestar personal typewriter. It runs on four D-size batteries and has a 6,000-word text memory and a self-contained printer that has never failed me.

Robert Ludlum: I have a little book I got from the state department called *Key Officers of Foreign Service Posts Guide for Business Representatives* that I always carry with me when I travel abroad. If you ever get into trouble, it lists all the ambassadors and deputies, their addresses and phone numbers. A one-year, two-issue subscription is available for $5 from the U.S. Government Printing Office, (202) 783-3238.

Roger Ebert, *film critic:* I use e-mail to send and receive messages when I am in my hotel room. When I need a hard copy of a document that I'm working on or that's stored on the

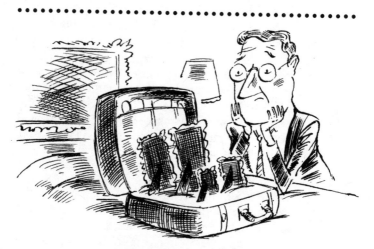

Heartbreak Hotel

Men are almost 50 percent more likely than women to be home-sick during extended business travel, according to a survey by the Marriott Corporation.

hard drive of my laptop, I just use MCI or CompuServe to send myself the document as a fax to my hotel's fax number, and then the hotel delivers the document right to my door—it sure beats carrying a portable printer.

Peter Vidmar, *Olympic gold medalist, TV sports commentator:* I use a Franklin Day Planner, and when I have a flight scheduled, I prioritize my tasks for that day with a "P" next to the items I can do on the plane. I don't feel pressured to get these things done before I leave, and I know I'll have plenty of time to complete them once in flight.

Howie Mandel, *comedian:* I always carry a laptop computer with me when I fly to cover stains caused by food I dropped during turbulence.

CLEARING CUSTOMS

Robert Ludlum: Declare everything at customs and when filling out your customs form, write very, very clearly in block letters.

Robin Cook: Don't buy anything in the duty-free shops. For the small amount of money you save on things like alcohol, it's not worth it. If you buy something overseas, ship it home.

BEATING JET LAG

Herschel Walker, *running back, Philadelphia Eagles professional football team:* After we land, I always go out for a good run. That and a shower make me feel like I'm starting my day all over.

Brian Boitano, *Olympic skating gold medalist:* There are these two pressure points I massage about four times during a flight. If you follow your collar bone across your neck and then down toward your sternum, there are two points in the corner on the inside where it makes a 90-degree angle, and I massage those while covering my belly button with my other hand. These pressure points are supposed to help you adjust to time differences and jet lag. I don't know if it really helps, but I don't ever want to not do it and find out.

Arnold Schwarzenegger, *actor:* I was in New York once when it was snowing outside and I only had 20 minutes. But I really needed some exercise. So I put my gym shorts on and ran up and down the hotel stairwell. When I came back I

● ●

SAVING MONEY

Look for new airlines, which compete harder for survival: Skybus, Family Air, Kiwi Airlines, Reno Air and Morris Air are a few.

▪ Go to discount ticket agencies (airfare consolidators) for the lowest ticket prices. Two such places are Travel Bargains at 1-800-872-8385 and Travel 800 at 1-800-359-2432. Look for others in the travel pages of your local newspaper.

▪ Shop around for better hotel prices. Hotel consolidators, similar to those for airfare, can track down the best rates for you. Two good services are the Hotel Reservations Network at 1-800-964-6835 and Quikbook at 1-800-221-3531, which cover most popular business destinations.

▪ Link air and ground frequent-flyer programs. Even if you're an infrequent flier, you can now earn air miles. The Marriott Miles program, for example, offers 500 frequent-flier miles on many major airlines when you stay a night at a Marriott hotel. To enroll, call 1-800-367-6453.

▪ Book early. Buying tickets in advance usually saves money. If the airline later drops the price, you can recover the difference.

● ●

dropped on the floor exhausted, but I had the greatest exercise! For free! With nothing—no machines, never left the hotel, and kept my appointment.

AT THE HOTEL

Mal Z. Lawrence, *comedian:* As soon as you get to your hotel, get on the phone and confirm your return trip.

Wayne Cotter, *comedian:* I always check out the TV to see if they have that movie deal with those soft-porn movies where you get five free minutes. I never actually pay for the movie, but I always watch the five-minute sample, and that's tricky because you have to time it out carefully so you don't just get the credits or five minutes of plot.

Ed McBain, *author*, Mary, Mary: I walk a lot, so one thing I always do in a strange city is ask the doorman of my hotel if there is anywhere I shouldn't go. I always preface the question by explaining that I'm from New York. I was in Denver last year, and when I asked the doorman of my hotel if there was anywhere I shouldn't walk, he said, "Well, I wouldn't walk four blocks to the right, because the Crips and the Bloods are fighting over drug territory there." Boy, was I glad I asked.

Robin Cook: If you are in a new city and want to find a good restaurant, the best place to ask is at a mom-and-pop bookstore. By far the best and most consistent tips have come from people who own small bookstores. This does not apply to chain bookstores.

Jay Leno, *host*, The Tonight Show: I usually pick restaurants not for the food but because I can keep my eye on my car and make sure the valet stays away from it.

Bernard Shaw, *anchor*, CNN PrimeNews: If you're in a new city and want to find a great restaurant, call the food editor of the local newspaper.

TIPS ON TIPPING

Joe Bob Briggs: I divide the world into five-dollar people and ten-dollar people. I ask myself, "What was this job worth? A five or a ten?" When I decide it's only a five, I usually feel guilty and go back and give 'em a ten anyway.

Brian Boitano: I'm really up front about it. I always ask my travel agent about it before I leave, or I ask the concierge of my hotel or the people at the desk, "Do you tip a percentage here, or is it included in the bill?" Tipping is different in every country you go to. I was just in Germany and tipping is more of a token there than anything else. No matter what the bill comes to, they just throw down a couple of marks.

Peter Arnett: I always carry a hundred U.S. dollars in single bills and distribute these at airports wherever I am, at the rate of one per bag or service.

Branford Marsalis: It's a dollar a bag—unless I'm late

for my flight, in which case it's ten dollars a bag, and I have them take it right to the plane.

Robert Ludlum: Don't ever worry about tipping with dollars, no matter what country you're in. Dollars are acceptable everywhere and preferable in many places.

YOUR PLANE IS DELAYED OR GROUNDED

Ed Perkins, editor of the *Consumer Reports Travel Letter:* If you're running late for a connecting flight, in the air, tell a flight attendant as soon as you realize you might have a problem. Sometimes they'll have a car waiting for you at the aircraft and not even take you through the main terminal. On the ground, run to the first person you find in uniform. Some of these customer service agents carry cellular phones at their sides, so they have a direct link to flights.

CANCELED FLIGHTS

Ed Perkins: Head for the pay phone and call the airline. You'll get faster service than if you get in a long line of other stranded travelers standing at the counter. If you have no luck with the airline, call your travel agent. He or she will be able to cope with your dilemma infinitely better than you will. Know your rights. You may be entitled to meals, lodging or free airfare or more, but it all depends on the circumstances. Get a copy of the Department of Transportation's booklet *Fly-Rights: A Guide to Air Travel in the U.S.* by writing to the Consumer Information Center, Department 131Z, Pueblo, CO 81009. Enclose a check or money order for $1 payable to Superintendent of Documents. Keep trying. If you don't get the answer you're looking for, ask someone else. Not all airline employees interpret the rules in the same way. If one's not helpful, just get in somebody else's line.

—Gregg Stebben

Part 10

ASK *MEN'S HEALTH*

20 Questions on Every Man's Mind

From socks to sweat to sex, here are some things that have guys puzzled.

• • • • • • • • • • • • • • • • • •

Here is just a smattering of the letters we received this past year at *Men's Health* magazine. We can't publish them all in the magazine, and we certainly can't print them all here. But these 20, I feel, do a pretty good job of representing the kinds of things on most men's minds.

—*Mike Lafavore*

SOCK UNCERTAINTY

Q. It happens at least twice a week. My wife stops me as I'm rushing out the door in the morning and tells me to change my socks because they don't go with what I'm wearing. What part of a man's clothing should they match?

—E. B., Newark, New Jersey

A. Your socks don't need to exactly match anything you're wearing, says G. Bruce Boyer, author of the book *Eminently Suitable*. Instead, your socks should be in the same color family as your trousers, but a shade darker or lighter. For example, dark gray suit? Wear lighter gray socks. Light tan suit? Wear darker tan socks. It's a simple rule with equally simple corollaries: Never wear a completely different color, such as brown socks with a navy blue suit; also, never wear black socks with anything other than a tuxedo.

PAIN IN THE RAIN

Q. My grandfather always told me he could predict rain with his "creaky old bones." I thought he was pulling my leg, but now it seems I have the same gift. About a year ago, I broke my ankle playing softball, and since then it gets sore whenever it's damp or raining. What gives?

—J. W., Alexandria, Virginia

A. As you've discovered, bones don't have to be old to be creaky. When a delicate joint like an ankle breaks, it may not heal perfectly. As a consequence, nerves are exposed along the jagged fault line. Down in these same spaces are microscopic air bubbles that are influenced by barometric pressure. When the air pressure outside drops quickly—a harbinger of wet weather—the air inside you expands. That change may stimulate the exposed nerve endings and cause the pain, says Kenneth Johnson, M.D., orthopedic surgeon with the Mayo Clinic in Scottsdale, Arizona. It's not just broken bones that are affected by weather. Anyone with a joint inflammation such as bursitis, tendinitis or arthritis is likely to become an amateur meteorologist.

GIVE ME AN X-LARGE

Q. I recently heard about a medical procedure that can enlarge a man's penis with cells taken from his abdomen. Is there really such an operation? Are there any risks?

—*W. W., Pleasantville, New Jersey*

A. Yes, a larger penis or, rather, a wider penis may be yours, if you really want it that badly. The procedure you refer to is called circumferential autologous penile engorgement (or CAPE, if you don't mind). It involves inserting a tube into the abdominal wall, vacuuming out fat cells and injecting them under the skin of the penis. It should be noted that CAPE—when it works—adds only girth, not length, to what nature gave you, says *Men's Health* magazine advisor Kenneth A. Goldberg, M.D., founder and director of the Male Health Center in Dallas. The result is a bit like having a penis with a spare tire around it. The extra layer of fat tends to make erections feel a bit mushy, we are told. There's also a risk that your penis will lose in sensitivity what it gains in circumference, and the risk that the added layer of fat will create a bumpy surface on the penis. "Since long-term results are still not known, we don't perform or endorse this procedure," says Dr. Goldberg.

IRON ARITHMETIC

Q. A lot of my workout buddies try to lift the most weight possible whenever we go to the gym. I usually just work with lighter weights since I'm just trying to stay toned, but I was wondering, what's the best way of finding out my maximum? Also, why isn't bench-pressing 100 pounds 20 times the same as pressing 200 pounds 10 times?

—*T. C., St. Louis, Missouri*

A. There are two ways to find out the maximum weight you can lift. The first way is simply to pile on the weights until you can't lift any more. Be sure to use a spotter, as the consequences of error here are fairly ugly. The other way is safer and requires only a pencil and paper. Figure that the amount you can lift 10 times is three-fourths of what you'd be able to lift once. Or the amount you can lift 20 times is three-fifths of what you'd be able to do once. For example, if you're capable of doing 10 repetitions at 100 pounds, your one-repetition maximum is about 135 pounds (100 divided by .75). If you're able to lift 100 pounds 20 times, your one-repetition maximum is likely to be close to 165 pounds (100 divided by .60).

The reason lifting 100 pounds 20 times isn't the same as lifting 200 pounds 10 times is that the intensity of the lift, and the effect on the muscle, isn't the same. As a general rule, heavier weights and lower repetitions do a better job of increasing muscle mass and strength. Strength is gained in the muscle by putting strain on it and breaking it down. The greater the strain, the greater the breakdown—and subsequent buildup.

SLIPPERY SEX

Q. My wife and I often use massages as foreplay, and inevitably our massage oil winds up doubling as a lubricant for sex. Can this cause any problem for either of us?

—*A. F., St. Louis, Missouri*

A. The massage oil shouldn't cause anything more serious than a minor irritation—unless you use condoms. Mineral oils and other oil-based lotions weaken latex condoms. Studies have shown that oil-based lubricants cause the layers of latex in a condom to separate, increasing the chance of breakage. By the way, you can't tell if a condom's weak by looking at it, says David J. Martin, Ph.D., a director of the HIV Infection Treatment Team at the Harbor-UCLA Medical Center in Torrance, California. To be on the safe side, use water-based lotions for your massage.

AFFAIR TURNED SOUR

Q. I'm 40 years old and have been married for 14 years. I had an affair with a female co-worker that got way out of hand. I ended it after a month, but we've been avoiding each other ever since. What's the best way to ease the tension in the office?

—*N. D., Boston, Massachusetts*

A. As with any wound, a severed romance takes time to heal. Because you broke off the affair, it is up to you to salvage the friendship. The first step is to be patient. Give her two to four weeks to get over the initial shock and anger. Meanwhile, if you happen to see her at the water cooler, don't avoid her or be overly friendly—just be yourself. After the cool-off period, you can try to talk to her about putting the affair behind you, but don't make a date to do this. "Drinks for two is probably what got you in trouble in the first place," says Karen Aronoff, a lecturer on organizational behavior at the University of Miami's School of Business Administration in Florida. If she doesn't want to talk, just continue to treat her cordially, as you would anyone else in the office, and try to put her out of your mind.

If the situation is interfering with your work, consider talking with your boss as a last resort. He or she might be able to create a little breathing room by reassigning one of you to another project or department.

TROUBLE IN THE SADDLE

Q. I do a lot of bike riding, about 60 miles per week. Lately, I've noticed a lessening of the pleasure in my orgasm and a decline in my ability to keep an erection during intercourse. Could the bike riding be causing my problems?
—*T. B., Minneapolis, Minnesota*

A. It's quite possible that your trouble in the saddle is caused by all those hours on the bike. What can happen from too much cycling is that the nerves under the penis, called the pudendal nerves, become compressed. Numbness can result and with repeated episodes of compression this could lead to reduced sensations and, in extreme cases, impotence.

Solving the problem may be as simple as adjusting the position of your seat. For example, if you cycle with the tip of your seat pointing upward, change it so it's exactly level (or at no more than a 5-degree incline).

Still not comfortable? A wider saddle may help alleviate the problem. Or ask your local bike shop about anatomical saddles or those with gel or some other form of extra cushioning, such as the Avocet GelFlex, about $30.

SWEDISH FOG

Q. Please answer once and for all what benefits there are in using steam rooms or saunas. I have heard that the high heat in saunas kills viruses that could cause colds. True?

—*D. M., Winchester, Virginia*

A. Steam rooms and saunas can help relax you by opening pores, loosening the connective tissues around your joints and muscles and generally relieving everyday tension. But most medical claims get fogged up when you look at them closely, says Robert Nirschl, M.D., medical director of the Virginia Sportsmedicine Institute in Arlington. There's no medical evidence that steam rooms or saunas kill viruses. Nor, for that matter, is there any medical evidence to support the popular beliefs that they stimulate weight loss, help clear up problem skin or cleanse toxins from the body.

DUMBBELL HELL

Q. I normally exercise in the morning before going to work. My routine consists of 20 to 25 minutes of dumbbell work as well as a session on Nautilus machines. Once in a while, I will play a half-hour of racquetball, too. Regardless of the length or type of workout, I usually end up having a headache for most of the day. What can I do about this?

—*H. G., Charlotte, North Carolina*

A. We know you're probably a little worried that there's something horribly wrong with you. Chances are, your headaches are nothing serious. There's even a name for them, exertional headaches, and, just as you describe, they're triggered by vigorous exercise. Any kind of physical exertion naturally raises blood pressure, which can have the added effect of increasing sinus pressure. In some people this brings on a headache, says Scott Haldeman, M.D., Ph.D., associate professor of neurology at the University of California, Irvine. Short, intense bouts of exercise are most likely to spark the problem, since they quickly boost blood pressure, heart rate and adrenaline levels in the bloodstream. One remedy, Dr. Haldeman says, is to scale back the intensity of your exercise. Another option is to take acetaminophen or aspirin 30 minutes before your workout to ward off the headache. If the headaches persist or if they become severe, stop exercising and see a physician immediately.

IS THIS ALL THERE IS?

Q. I have the desire. I have the erection. What I don't have is any sensation when I climax. I know it's happening, but there are no fireworks. This is scary.

—D. C., Baltimore, Maryland

A. This sounds like something you should talk to your doctor about. There are a number of possible causes for your condition. Some drugs, particularly antidepressants or blood pressure medications, can mute the sensation of orgasm. Your situation could also be linked to your state of mind between the sheets, says Irwin Goldstein, M.D., professor of urology at Boston University School of Medicine. If sex is turned into a performance sport, if things have become old hat with your partner or if you're under a heap of stress, your orgasms could be suffering in the way you describe. If so, don't delay; get to a couples counselor. Another cause could be nerve damage, which is sometimes sustained during an operation on the prostate. If you'd had such an operation, you'd probably already know the potential consequences.

EXPOSED ROOTS

Q. I am 39 and my gums have begun to recede slightly and slowly during the last two years. This has exposed some root area, making my teeth temperature- and pressure-sensitive. What can I do to keep the recession and root exposure from continuing?

—J. F., Medford, New Jersey

A. What's happening to your gums is a natural consequence of aging, if that makes you feel any better. The good news is there've been tremendous developments in stopping, even reversing, gum damage, says Michael G. Newman, D.D.S., president of the American Academy of Periodontology. To avoid aggravating the problem, he suggests, brush only up and down and use a soft-bristle brush. Also, switch to toothpastes containing potassium nitrate (Denquel and Sensodyne-F), which slow down nerve impulses in the teeth. For deeper recessions, ask your dentist about bonding agents to fill the space. At a certain point, though, you'll be looking at gum surgery. Most procedures can be performed in a dentist's office in under an hour and cost between $300 and $1,000.

LIFE'S A DRAG

Q. I'm 32 years old and constantly tired. I blame it on having had mononucleosis when I was 16. I don't feel as if I have ever gotten it out of my system. I would like to have more energy, feel less tired, sleep less and just feel good. What can I do?

—*M. C., Madison, Wisconsin*

A. It's highly unlikely that you're still sick from that same case of mononucleosis, but there are numerous other factors that could account for your fatigue. David N. Neubauer, M.D., associate director of the Johns Hopkins Sleep Disorders Center in Baltimore, suggests that you take a look at your lifestyle. If you sit at a desk all day and on the couch all evening, you may have unintentionally set your engine at a low idle. Make at least a small commitment to exercise—even just to walk up the stairs at work for starters—and see if you don't begin to feel more energized. Second, even though you say you sleep a lot, you may have a sleep disorder that's preventing you from getting any real rest. To check this and to rule out other medical problems, ask your doctor for a full physical exam.

INSTANT FAMILY

Q. My longtime girlfriend has two children. I always figured that was no problem. They were hers, not mine. Then she and I decided to get married, which is a little like stepping off a cliff in the best of circumstances. What can I do to make it easier?

—*F. R., Lexington, Kentucky*

A. It would be a mistake to attack this as a who's-the-boss problem, says John Visher, M.D., psychiatrist and co-founder of the

Stepfamily Association of America. In fact, you can't treat this as a problem at all. Problems need solutions, and what you need right now is all the patience you can muster for a necessarily slow adjustment period.

"It's important not to just thrust the new family situation at the kids," says Dr. Visher. Rule of thumb: Expect it to take up to a year building rapport with a child who is six or under and even longer for an older child. The key to rapport is trust. Dr. Visher offers these suggestions.

- Become a friend first. Schedule some time together for activities such as playing miniature golf or going fishing or skiing or visiting a zoo.

- Find a new home as soon as possible. This way, you won't feel like you're constantly crossing boundaries and invading the children's spaces.

- Go easy on the discipline. "Many guys come in thinking their job is to start acting like a parent right away, but this just strains an already tough situation," says Dr. Visher.

- Don't insist on being called "Dad." That title may come in time. Meanwhile, though, demanding it as you walk in the door is likely to breed resentment. To the children it's a direct challenge to their own father.

- Don't cross the ex. Whatever you may think of their father, don't say disparaging things about him. "That comes across as rejecting part of them," says Dr. Visher.

JUNK-FOOD JUNKIE

Q. I'm in great shape and I love sports. But I also have a weakness for junk food. Candy, cheeseburgers, cookies, cake, you name it. Tell me one good reason why I should give it up.

—*T. S., Denver, Colorado*

A. We're going to surprise you. We're not going to tell you to give up junk food. The stuff won't make you fat as long as you keep exercising away the extra calories. Nor will it dull your competitive edge as long as you're getting the essential nutrients you need from other foods. Take world-class runner Bill Rodgers, for example. He managed to secure several world medals despite having a love of junk food.

It's when cookies and candy start replacing healthful food in your diet and you fail to work off those fatty treats that you'll see a decline in your athletic powers. The key is to try to limit your fat calories to no more than 25 percent of your daily intake. You can have your cake and still reach this diet goal by making some rather painless substitutions for your high-fat habit. Eat dried fruit rolls for your candy fix. Top lean burgers with low-fat Swiss instead of cheddar, and try out some of those low-fat or nonfat cookies and cakes made by Pepperidge Farms, R.W. Frookies and Entenmann's.

IN SEARCH OF COOL

Q. I sweat. I mean *really* sweat, even when I'm sitting around. I know the body is supposed to be 70 percent water, but it seems like I have more than my share. What's wrong? What can I do about it?

—*G. F., San Jose, California*

A. One way to ensure that your sweat glands keep you clammy is to worry about them. Stress triggers the body circuitry and causes you to perspire more. So first of all, don't concern yourself too much over this. If it helps, remember that perspiring is an essential body function, required to keep the body cool.

Okay, you want better advice. If you're constantly drenched, we don't blame you. Some men don't just sweat rivulets, they sweat rivers, all on account of a rare little glitch in the central nervous system known as hyperhidrosis. In effect, if you imagine that sweat glands have a dial from 1 to 10 controlling their output, men with this condition are always pumping out a 10. Stephen Smith, M.D., a dermatologist at the University of Louisville School of Medicine, tenders hope in the form of prescription antiperspirants, which are much stronger than the kind you see advertised on TV. If that route doesn't lead anywhere, you'll have to take the wrap—medicated wrap, that is, and apply it to the offending zones once or twice a week. Over time the medicine in the wraps shuts down the perspiring glands and leads you back to dry land.

CAN VITAMINS CURE HIVES?

Q. Starting last November, I've been taking vitamins in doses higher than the recommended dietary allowance. Since then, I've been getting hives. Why is this happening? Could I have an allergic reaction to the vitamins?

—*E. P., Canton, Ohio*

A. Chances are, you're not allergic to the vitamins themselves, but you may be allergic to one or more of the additives in the products, says Jeffrey Blumberg, Ph.D., associate director/senior scientist and chief of the antioxidants research laboratory at the U.S. Department of Agriculture Human Nutrition Research Center of Aging at Tufts University in Medford, Massachusetts. Check the label for food colorings, starches, dyes, stabilizers or preservatives, any of which could be the culprit. Skip the vitamins for a couple of weeks to see if the rash disappears. If it does, then switch to a brand of vitamins that has no additives. If the problem persists, see an allergist or dermatologist. There are dozens of other things that might be causing your hives.

CRABBY WIFE

Q. Last week my wife and I discovered she had crabs. And I'm not talking about the kind you order at Red Lobster. I found this upsetting, to say the least, since I am not infested. She assures me she hasn't been unfaithful. Is it possible the critters weren't sexually transmitted?

—*S. R., Laramie, Wyoming*

A. Yes, it is. Pubic lice (blood-feasting insects, which, under a magnifying glass, do bear a close resemblance to teeny-tiny crabs) are easily picked up from towels, bed sheets, clothes, even that funky sofa you bought at the yard sale. It doesn't take body-to-body contact to pass the little guys around, since they can live away from a host for up to 24 hours and their eggs can survive for several days. So, for example, your wife could have had the bad luck to have used a towel at her health club that had not been washed in hot enough water and picked up pubic lice from an infested exerciser who used the towel the day before.

Crabs itch like crazy, but healthwise, they're no big deal. Most cases can be treated with over-the-counter products, such as RID, Nix or A-200 Pyrinate, or with a prescription medicine called Kwell.

HAPPY FEET

Q. I'm suffering from sock confusion. I've read that polypropylene socks are the best for sports, but I've also seen ads claiming acrylic socks are preferred by pro athletes. When I go shopping, nearly all the socks are cotton. Is there really a difference?

—*S. G., Renton, Washington*

A. When it comes to sports socks, cotton's no good—it soaks up sweat, holds the wetness and rubs against your skin, causing blisters and, in the winter, cold feet.

Acrylic and polypropylene, on the other hand, are both good choices, says Dave Getchell, equipment editor for *Backpacker* magazine. That's because these two man-made fibers wick sweat away from skin. Which one to choose is up to you. Acrylic is softer and less scratchy than poly; it cushions your feet better when playing hoops or other high-impact sports, but doesn't get rid of moisture quite as well. So if you sweat like a boiler man, go with poly.

Don't forget wool socks. They're the warmest for long winter jaunts in the woods. If you break out in hives at the mention of wool, try wearing a thin poly liner inside the wool sock to avoid skin contact.

THE JACK SPRAT DIET

Q. I've read plenty of articles on cutting back on fat, and I have to ask: Is it possible to cut back too far? Is there a point of diminishing returns, or are there any possible side effects of low-fat diets?

—*N. F. B., Farmington Hills, Michigan*

A. A certain small percentage of dietary fat is necessary to keep your body supplied with essential fatty acids, says Lynne Scott, R.D., director of the Diet Modification Clinic at Baylor College of Medicine in Houston. It would be almost impossible to lower your fat intake to the point where your body might suffer, she says. The only reported cases of fat deficiency come from people on long-term intravenous feedings. Nice try, though. "Hey, my body needs the extra-cheese-and-sausage deep dish!"

THE POST-COITAL COMA

Q. What makes a man feel weak and tired after ejaculation?
—*E. B., Lewisburg, Tennessee*

A. Two things. First, if you knock yourself out physically, it's bound to tucker you, whether it's from passionate lovemaking or a lambada marathon. Second, after a release of tension, it's natural to get a deep feeling of relaxation. The pelvic muscles become five to ten times more tense than normal when sexual arousal begins. After orgasm, this muscle tension drops to a level below where it began.

A lot depends on your baseline energy. If you sledge rocks all day, then stagger home for a quickie, the sudden relaxation might plunge you into the Z-zone. Try not to view it as a problem. Just enjoy the relaxation.

On the other hand, if you find you always sag into a coma after a romp in the sack no matter what you did that day, you're probably way out of shape. Take it as a message from your body that it's time to get fit.

Index

Note: <u>Underscored</u> page references indicate boxed text.
Boldface references indicate tables.